PITUITARY DISEASES

Edited by **Fawaz Assaad, Hansdetlef Wassmann** and **Maher Khodor**

Pituitary Diseases
http://dx.doi.org/10.5772/intechopen.72984
Edited by Fawaz Assaad, Hansdetlef Wassmann and Maher Khodor

Contributors

Mauro Bozzola, Chiara Montalbano, Elena Bozzola, Filomena Stamati, Daniela Larizza, Pietro Ferrara, Alberto Villani, Mario Francesco Fraioli, Andrea Pagano, Bernardo Fraioli, Pierpaolo Lunardi, Wafa Alaya, Manel Jemel, Fadia Boubaker, Olfa Berriche, Baha Zantour, Arwa Azmeh, Dorian Chauvet, Stephane Hans, Raydeh Al Khani, Fawaz Assaad

First published in London, United Kingdom, 2019 by IntechOpen
IntechOpen is the global imprint of INTECHOPEN LIMITED, registered in England and Wales, registration number: 11086078, The Shard, 25th floor, 32 London Bridge Street
London, SE19SG – United Kingdom
Printed in Croatia

British Library Cataloguing-in-Publication Data
A catalogue record for this book is available from the British Library

Additional hard copies can be obtained from orders@intechopen.com

Pituitary Diseases, Edited by Fawaz Assaad, Hansdetlef Wassmann and Maher Khodor
p. cm.
Print ISBN 978-1-78985-747-4
Online ISBN 978-1-78985-748-1

For EU product safety concerns :
IN TECH d.o.o., Prolaz Marije Krucifikse Kozulić 3, 51000 Rijeka, Croatia,
info@intechopen.com or visit our website at intechopen.com.

Meet the editors

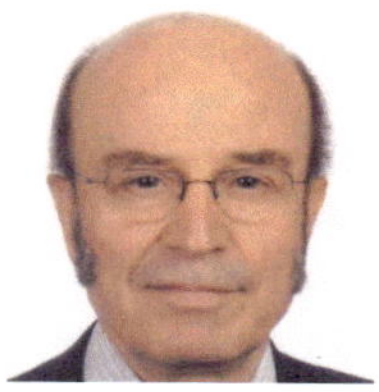

Professor Dr. Fawaz Assaad is a German Board-certified Neurosurgeon (Friedrich-Wilhelm University in Bonn, Germany), with over 30 years' experience in Neurosurgery and Neuroanatomy. He was the former head of the Neurosurgical Department at Damascus University, former team leader for the National Plan of Development Program and Curricula for the School of Medicine in Damascus University, Syria, former dean of the Medical School at Damascus University, Syria. He has also been the former Adjunct Professor at the Lebanese American University of Beirut, Lebanon and he was the founder of the Syrian Centre for Conservative and Surgical Treatment of Epilepsy in collaboration with Friedrich-Wilhelm University in Bonn, Germany. He is the senior consultant at neurosurgical departments in Germany and recently started working in research and running his own private clinic. His scientific efforts and research include: conservative and surgical spine therapy, hypophysis disease, stereotactic and functional neurosurgery, and conservative and surgical treatment of epilepsy.Professor Assaad has 15 published papers in international medical journals, is the author and editor of six books on neurosurgery and neuroanatomy, is supervisor of 23 postgraduate MSc theses, and has more than 65 presentations, lectures, and symposiums.

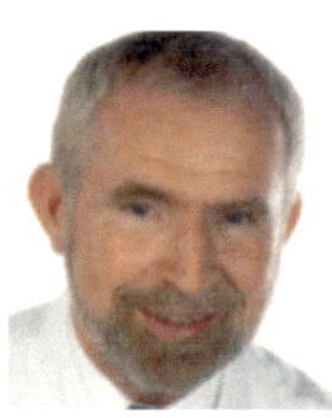

Professor Dr. Med. Hansdetlef Wassmann was appointed in 1988 as a professor in neurosurgery at the University-Klinik of Bonn, Germany. In 1977 he attained a specialist's qualification certificate in neurosurgery. He graduated in 1970 from the Medical College, University of Bonn, Heidelberg, and Vienna. He was a former chief of the Department of Neurosurgery, University-Klinik of Muenster, Germany. His scientific efforts and research projects include: microneurosurgical therapy of cerebrovascular diseases, including experimental and clinical studies on hyperbaric oxygenation in cerebral hypoxia, clinical and experimental investigation of brain infarction and cerebral blood flow measurement, development of combined operative/interventional neuroradiological/open angioplasty procedures andobstructive vascular lesions and since 1994 intraoperative radiation therapy for cerebral malignant gliomas, including interstitial laser radiation of glioma and frameless stereotactic navigation. In 1995 he was involved in experimental research of "brain protective measurement" in transient intraoperative cerebral ischemia.

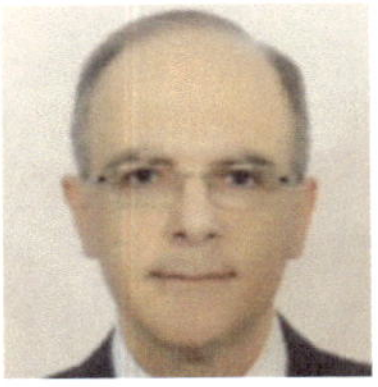

Professor Maher Khodor has been an American Board-certified internist since 1993. He attained ABIM certification in endocrinology, diabetes, and metabolism in 1995. He graduated from Maulana Azad Medical College in Delhi University, India, in 1988. He has been an associate professor and attending internist and endocrinologist at Damascus University Hospital, Faculty of Medicine, since 2000. His scientific efforts and research projects include: participation in the prospective study of the use of complementary activation products to monitor patients with systemic lupus erythematosus, participation in a randomized parallel study on the effect of theophylline as a loading dose in the emergency room in reducing the hospital stay of asthmatic patients, and participation in a multicenter randomized, double-blind, placebo-controlled trial on the effect of Orlistat in obese patients with noninsulin-dependent diabetes mellitus (later marketed as Xenical).

Contents

Preface

Dedication: To my beloved country, Syria, and to the first teacher, President Bashar Al-Assad, The Patron of science and scientists.

To the glowing University of Damascus, where I started my scientific career and where I spent the most beautiful twenty five years of my life.

Pituitary adenomas are the third most common intracranial neoplasms in adults, accounting for about 10% of all intracranial tumors. The age-adjusted incidence rate is 2.6 (2.6-2.8) cases per 100, 000. They are diagnosed when patients present with hormone hypersecretion, plus visual and neurologic deficits and hypopituitarism as a result of mass effect. They may also be found as pituitary incidentalomas. Pituitary adenomas that are gonadotroph adenomas are referred to as clinically nonfunctional adenomas (CNFPAs). CNFPAs and prolactinomas are the two most prevalent pituitary adenomas. This book presents seven chapters ranging from dedicated surgical technique for huge pituitary adenomas to management of celiac patients with growth failure, pituitary apoplexy, neuro ophthalmology findings, immunohistochemical studies, and transoral robotic surgery (TORS) with the da Vinci system.

The chapter entitled "Huge Pituitary Adenomas: Dedicated Surgical Technique and Indications for Extent of Tumour Removal in the Modern Era" explains a modified transsphenoidal technique to remove huge pituitary adenomas with marked suprasellar extension. The technique avoided the occurrence of a precocious descent of the suprasellar cisternal plane into the sellar plane during tumor removal and its related dangerous consequences. Comparing the results to similar patients operated on by the same authors using a standard surgical technique, we observed that total removal was accomplished in 64% of patients treated with the modified technique than 45% of patients treated with the standard transsphenoidal surgery. Moreover, better results were achieved concerning intraoperative CSF leak, postoperative CSF fistula, and average time of postoperative stay in hospital.

The next chapter is entiteld "Transoral Robotic Surgery Applied to the Skull Base" and herein the author describes a new and advanced method for transoral robotic surgery to reach the sellar and especially the pituitary tumors. For many years, robotic surgery with the da Vinci system (Intuitive Surgical Inc, Sunnyvale, CA, USA) has been increasingly adopted, especially in urology and gynecology. The beginning was with clear explanation of anatomy and cad cadaveric study as well as radiological study especially using computer tomography to explain the measurements and the procedure steps, afterwards the clinical studies during operation and the complications and difficulties, especially for solid pituitary tumors. This is an evolution in robotic neurosurgery for the future. From this innovative TORS for sellar tumors, we can emphasize some promising results on cystic tumors, in a minimally invasive perspective because the side effects were minor and transient. The 3D visualization is very good and the maneuverability of the robotic instruments is satisfying, even in narrow spaces.

Further on, the chapter "Management of Celiac Patients with Growth Failure" is a review article about growth failure in pediatric patients with celiac disease who fail to show acceleration of growth after a gluten-free diet. It defines celiac disease and its relation to growth hormone deficiency and other endocrinopathies of an autoimmune nature affecting the thyroid, adrenals, and gonads. Afterwards the author details the diagnostic criteria for GH deficiency, using multiple laboratory approaches, and emphasizes the relation to puberty where GH response to stimulatory testing may vary before and after the start of puberty. Finally, there is a description of the treatment and dosage of recombinant human GH, duration of treatment, and results on growth velocity. The author asserts that these are similar in both celiac disease patients on a strict gluten-free diet and in idiopathic GH deficiency children. It is an excellent well written review, with ample evidence based on scientific content and presented in simple language for the pediatrician and endocrinologist.

"Pituitary Apoplexy" is a very well written and interesting chapter. Pituitary tumor apoplexy (PA) is an uncommon acute clinical syndrome and one of the rare problems that is diagnostically and therapeutically challenging. It is frequently the onset of unknown pre-existing pituitary adenoma. The clinical spectrum of presentation does vary, but is often reserved only for classical presentation in contrast to "silent, subclinical or asymptomatic pituitary tumor apoplexy" even though the latter is the more frequent entity. Pituitary tumor apoplexy appears to be rare. The true incidence and prevalence of PA is difficult to establish either because the majority of the studies are retrospectives or because the diagnosis of PA is usually misdiagnosed and simply identified at surgery or during radiological investigation or pathological examination. According to the main retrospective series, an estimated prevalence of 6.2 cases per 100,000 inhabitants and an incidence of 0.17 episodes per 100,000 person-years were reported.

The outcome of acute apoplexy is variable and remains difficult to predict. A regular input and follow up from multidisciplinary team including neurosurgeons, endocrinologists, neuro-ophthalmologists, neuroradiologists, and neurologists is mandatory.

"Neuro-Ophthalmology Findings in Pituitary Disease " is chapter based on an important review of the literature about visual symptoms accompanying pituitary diseases. Pituitary tumors may compress surrounding structures such as optic chiasm leading to visual field defects including bitemporal hemianopia and visual disturbance. Chiasmal syndromes most commonly occur secondary to pituitary adenomas, craniopharyngiomas, meningiomas, and pituitary apoplexy. They may also compress cranial nerves III, IV, and VI, leading to ocular motility abnormalities. Pituitary adenomas are the most common cause of chiasmal compression. Patients with non-secreting tumors present initially with vision loss and these tumors can reach large sizes without causing other symptoms; however, hormonally active tumors are detected before vision loss because of systemic symptoms. Acute hemorrhage or infarction of the pituitary tumor known as pituitary apoplexy causes diplopia, loss of vision and visual field. Thus, the ophthalmologist role is crucial in diagnosis and treatment of pituitary tumors. As visual loss may be the first sign of recurrence after treatment, it is essential to repeat visual field and visual acuity testing every 6-12 months.

The last chapter "Hormone Secretion in Pituitary Adenomas:Immunohistochemical Studies" is a very interesting and valuable discussion on the classification of pituitary adenomas because various types of hormones, prehormonal substances, and transcription factors are detected in pituitary adenomas. Monohormonal secretion in pituitary adenomas is frequent; notably prolactin secretion. Bihormonal secretion is well known, classically GH-PRL and FSH-LH. Other combinations of bihormonal secretion are reported and these are sometimes underestimated. Plurihormonal secretion in pituitary adenomas is usually underestimated; it is in most cases subclinical. Immunohistochemical study of all pituitary hormones and pre-hormonal substances, as demonstrated by transcription factors, is not always available and it is frequently not performed. This chapter aims to clarify this underestimated and vague area of pituitary adenomas and to show the importance of immunohistochemical studies in the diagnosis and prediction of clinical outcomes of these adenomas. These adenomas reveal various histopathological patterns and tinctorial properties that prove to be unreliable and do not always correlate with the functional or immunohistochemical finding.

Fawaz Assaad (Editor)
Professor of Neurosurgery at Damascus University
School of Medicine
Damascus, Syria

Hansdetlef Wassmann (Co-editor)
Univ. Professor of Neurosurgery
former Director of the University Klinikum Muenster
Muenster, Germany

Maher Kodor (Co-editor)
Associate Professor of Endocrinology at Tartous University
School of Medicine
Damascus, Syria

Section 1

Introduction

Chapter 1

Introductory Chapter: Introduction to Pituitary Disease Management

Fawaz Assaad

Additional information is available at the end of the chapter

http://dx.doi.org/10.5772/intechopen.82295

1. Introduction

Pituitary diseases are serious systemic condition reported most likely in patients with an adenoma of the pituitary gland because of systemic changes resulting from hyper- or hypofunction of the pituitary gland. Both medical and surgical treatments have been used in the last decades; however, the prediction of post medical and postsurgical treatment is still controversial, even though different criteria for a cure have been suggested, especially the relationship between these criteria and the long-term control of the disease [1–3].

The current main treatment options available for pituitary diseases are transsphenoidal microsurgical surgery, medical treatment, and radiotherapy. Surgical outcome depends on the expertise of the surgeon, tumor size, and extension of the adenoma. Despite surgical removal is still the main treatment of pituitary adenomas; however, some patients are not cured by surgical treatment and need additional interventions. The main aim of treatment is to remove the tumor mass, control the disease by suppressing hormone hyperactivity to normal values, reduce morbidity and mortality (especially in acromegaly and Cushing's patients), and eliminate secondary comorbid complications. Such control may be achieved through either single or combined surgery, radiotherapy, and/or medical treatment. Continuous and long-term monitoring of the disease activity postoperatively, post medical treatment, or post radiotherapy is of high priority. However, the prediction of postoperative disease activity is a major challenge, and even though different criteria for a cure have been suggested, the relationship between these criteria and long-term disease control is still controversial. Morbidity and mortality rates in untreated and uncontrolled patients are very high due to the effect of raised hormone as well as the mass effect in the macroadenomas. Effective and aggressive long-term treatment is needed in some cases to normalize these rates. Delay in diagnosis and subsequent comorbidities are the main factors influencing the prognosis [3–8].

Several consensus documents have been published on various aspects of pituitary disease management. In the last 20 years, there is a consensus group in each kind of pituitary adenoma that reevaluates and updates the guidelines on criteria for cure. One of the important problems is the lack of reliable assays, assay standardization, and adequate normative data, which are major issues in the interpretation of these biochemical measures; especially these factors can lead to major discrepancies in the values obtained in different laboratories [9–12].

The reasons for the heterogeneity among hormone immunoassay results include variable calibration, epitope specificity of the chosen antibody, and differences in the specificity of antibody recognition of different hormone isoforms circulating in the serum. As a first step to improving the interpretation of GH assays, it is strongly recommended that the World Health Organization (WHO) international standard (WHO IS 98/574) be used, and the results be expressed in mass units (micrograms per liter) [13, 14].

This book provides detailed update on current diagnostic and therapeutic techniques useful in the management of pituitary diseases. The contents reflect the multidisciplinary approach needed for patients with pituitary diseases with contribution from neurosurgeons, endocrinologists, neurologists, radiologists, ophthalmologists, pathologists, and radiation oncologists. The book focuses on some pituitary diseases especially the most controversial subjects in the medical and surgical treatment like dedicated surgical technique by huge pituitary adenomas; moreover there is a special chapter about transoral robotic surgery (TORS) with the da Vinci system, other important subjects such as management of celiac patients with growth failure, pituitary apoplexy, neuro-ophthalmology findings in pituitary disease, and hormone secretion in pituitary adenomas: immunohistochemical studies.

Author details

Fawaz Assaad

Address all correspondence to: fawaz.assaad99@gmail.com

School of Medicine, Damascus University, Syria

References

[1] Roelfsema F, Biermasz NR, Pereira AM. Clinical factors involved in the recurrence of pituitary adenomas after surgical remission: A structured review and meta-analysis. Pituitary. 2012;**15**(1):71-83

[2] Buchfelder M, Schlaffer S. Surgical treatment of pituitary tumours. Best Practice & Research. Clinical Endocrinology & Metabolism. 2009;**23**(5):677-692

[3] Ciric I, Ragin A, Baumgartner C, Pierce D. Complications of transsphenoidal surgery: Results of a national survey, review of the literature, and personal experience. Neurosurgery. 1997;**40**:225-236

[4] Giustina A, Chanson P, Bronstein MD, Klibanski A, Lamberts S, Casanueva FF, et al. A consensus on criteria for cure of acromegaly. The Journal of Clinical Endocrinology and Metabolism. 2010;**95**:3141-3148

[5] Beauregard C, Truong U, Hardy J, Serri O. Long-term outcome and mortality after transsphenoidal adenomectomy. Clinical Endocrinology. 2003;**58**(1):86-91. PubMed PMID: 12519417

[6] Caron P, Morange-Ramos I, Cogne M, Jaquet P. Three-year follow-up of acromegalic patients treated with intramuscular slow-release lanreotide. The Journal of Clinical Endocrinology and Metabolism. 1997;**82**:18-22

[7] Barkan AL, Halasz I, Dornfeld KJ, et al. Pituitary irradiation is ineffective in normalizing plasma insulin-like growth factor I in patients with acromegaly. The Journal of Clinical Endocrinology. 1997;**82**:3187-3191

[8] Landolt AM, Haller D, Lomax N, et al. Stereotactic radiosurgery for recurrent surgically treated adenomas. comparison with fractionated radiotherapy. Journal of Neurosurgery. 1998;**88**:1002-1008

[9] Colao A, Pivonello R, Auriem RS, Briganti F, Galdiero M, Tortora F, et al. Predictors of tumor shrinkage after primary therapy with somatostatin analogs in acromegaly: A prospective study in 99 patients. The Journal of Clinical Endocrinology and Metabolism. 2006;**91**:2112-2118

[10] Cozzi R, Montini M, Attanasio R, Albizzi M, Lasio G, Lodrini S, et al. Primary treatment of acromegaly with octreotide LAR: A long-term (up to nine years) prospective study of its efficacy in the control of disease activity and tumor shrinkage. The Journal of Clinical Endocrinology and Metabolism. 2006;**91**:1397-1403

[11] Melmed S, Sternberg R, Cook D, Klibanski A, Chanson P, Bonert V, et al. A critical analysis of pituitary tumor shrinkage during primary medical therapy in acromegaly. The Journal of Clinical Endocrinology and Metabolism. 2005;**90**:4405-4410

[12] Amato G, Mazziotti G, Rotondi M, Iorio S, Doga M, Sorvillo F, et al. Long-term effects of lanreotide SR and octreotide LAR on tumour shrinkage and GH hypersecretion in patients with previously untreated acromegaly. Clinical Endocrinology. 2002;**56**:65-71

[13] Bidlingmaier M. Problems with GH assays and strategies toward standardization. European Journal of Endocrinology. 2008;**159**(Suppl. 1):S41-S44

[14] Trainer PJ, Barth J, Sturgeon C, Wieringaon G. Consensus statement on the standardisation of GH assays. European Journal of Endocrinology. 2006;**155**:1-2

Section 2

Surgical Management

Chapter 2

Huge Pituitary Adenomas: Dedicated Surgical Technique and Indications for Extent of Tumour Removal in the Modern Era

Mario Francesco Fraioli, Andrea Pagano,
Bernardo Fraioli and Pierpaolo Lunardi

Additional information is available at the end of the chapter

http://dx.doi.org/10.5772/intechopen.77269

Abstract

Transsphenoidal surgery is the most indicated approach not only for small and large pituitary adenomas but also for huge ones. A modified transsphenoidal technique to remove huge pituitary adenomas with marked suprasellar extension (4–8 cm of maximum diameter) resulted very useful in authors' experience. The technique allowed avoiding the occurrence of a precocious descent of the suprasellar cisternal plane into the sellar plane during tumor removal and its related dangerous consequences. Technique was performed opening at the beginning only the lateral parts of peritumoral dura mater, and after removal of lateral parts of the tumor, the central part of peritumoral dura mater was opened and the central intrasellar and suprasellar parts of the tumor were removed. Comparing the results to similar patients operated by the same authors with standard surgical technique, we observed that total removal was accomplished in 64% of patients treated with modified technique than 45% of patients treated with standard transsphenoidal surgery. Moreover, better results were achieved concerning intraoperative CSF leak, postoperative CSF fistula, and average time of postoperative stay in hospital. For invasive dumbbell-shaped pituitary adenomas, particular therapeutic plans are necessary.

Keywords: pituitary adenoma, transsphenoidal surgery, cerebrospinal fluid fistula, huge adenomas, cranial base reconstruction

1. Introduction

Voluminous pituitary adenomas with marked suprasellar extension can be effectively treated by transsphenoidal surgery [1], except for rare cases in which transcranial approach should be performed [2]. Regardless tumor size, invasive or noninvasive behavior of the adenoma is a crucial factor that influences extent of tumor removal. Huge noninvasive pituitary adenomas are extra-arachnoid tumors, compressing and displacing suprasellar nervous and vascular structures, and adequate surgical technique allows total or gross total removal avoiding complications (intraoperative cerebrospinal fluid fistula, vascular damages, etc.). On the other hand, invasive dumbbell-shaped tumors pass through diaphragm sellae and arachnoid membrane without compressing or displacing but encasing vascular and nervous structures. Removal of suprasellar portions of these last tumors is very dangerous because critical structures are encountered before suprasellar portion of the tumor, differently from noninvasive tumors, which displace neurovascular structures above the tumor.

2. Main body

Out of more than 1400 pituitary adenomas operated on in our institute (by Bernardo Fraioli, Chief of Department of Neurosurgery 1991–2014 and Mario F Fraioli, Professor of Neurosurgery, University of Rome "TorVergata") from 1993 to 2015, we selected 138 patients operated from 2005 to 2015 for huge pituitary adenoma with marked suprasellar extension (sized 4–7.5 cm of max. diam.).

2.1. Patients population and clinical data

Patients' age was between 17 and 81 years, with average age of 54.4 years; 77 were female and 61 male. All patients presented visual disturbances, consisting in bitemporal hemianopsia in all ones, visual acuity deficit in 103 patients, and abducens and oculomotor nerve palsy in 11 and 5 patients, respectively. Symptomatic hypopituitarism was registered in 69 patients, while subclinical hormonal deficits were discovered in other 45 patients; these last patients were treated with substitutive hormonal therapy before and after surgery. Normal hormonal status, although if corresponding to the inferior limits of the normal reference range, was evident in the other 24 patients.

2.2. MR tumors characteristics

At preoperative MRI, enlargement of sella turcica and suprasellar extension was present in all tumors; prevalent median extension was present in 121, while lateral extension into the temporal lobe was evident in 12 and anterior frontal extension in 5 patients; in 127 patients, optic chiasm was above displaced, while in the other 11, it was encased into the tumor. A1 tracts of anterior cerebral arteries were superiorly and laterally displaced (**Figure 1**) in 131, while in the other 7 patients, they were encased in the tumor (**Figures 2** and **3**). Unilateral and bilateral cavernous sinus invasion were evident in 39 and 6 adenomas, respectively. In invasive tumors, angio-MR images show normal position of A1 tracts of anterior cerebral arteries (**Figure 2**), differently from huge noninvasive adenomas which cause displacement of vascular (**Figure 1**) and nervous structures.

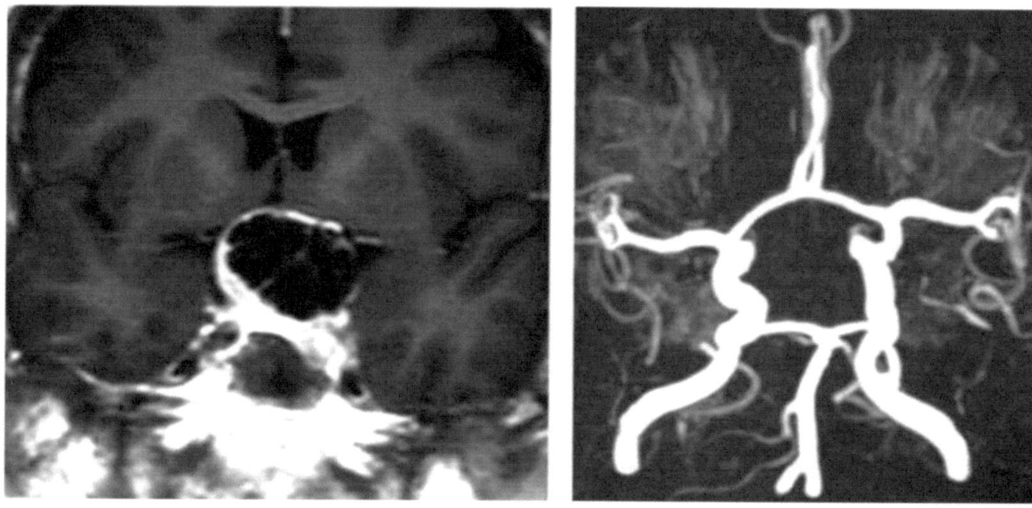

Figure 1. Invasive voluminous hemorrhagic noninvasive pituitary adenoma. Angio-MR image shows superior displacement of A1 tracts of anterior cerebral arteries.

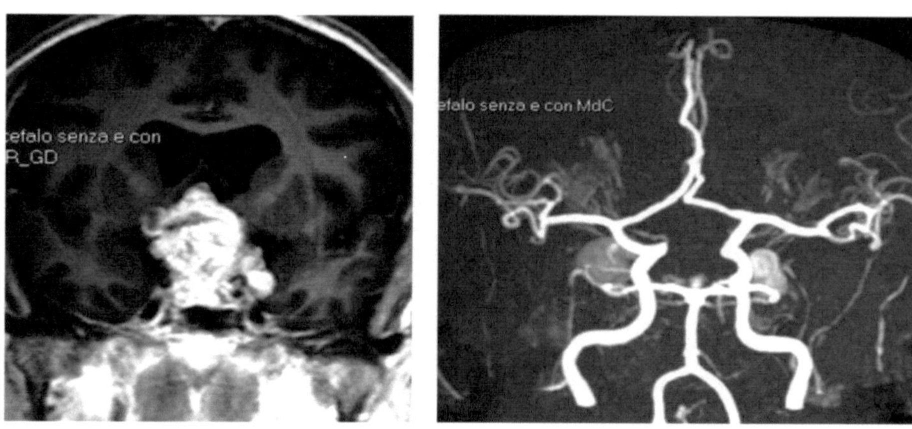

Figure 2. Invasive pituitary macroadenoma with marked suprasellar extension. Angio-MR image shows normal position of A1 tracts of anterior cerebral arteries.

2.3. Therapeutic strategy

Considering that adenomas of this series were invasive, and of large size, our therapeutic strategy was to remove tumor as most as possible, avoiding to remove invasive tumoral component strictly connected to crucial neurovascular structures, which are often encased into the tumor; hazardous maneuvers were avoided, such as other authors reported for other benign tumors of sellar-suprasellar compartment [3]. In the cases of huge invasive adenomas with involvement of optic chiasm, A1 tracts of anterior cerebral arteries and diencephalus crossed the tumors and

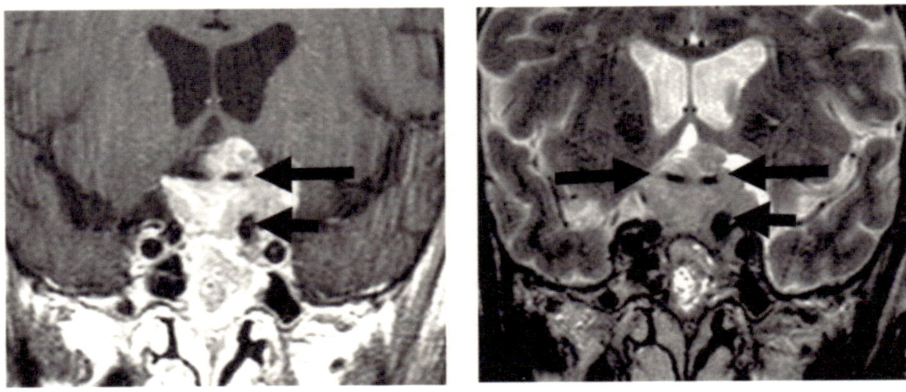

Figure 3. Invasive pituitary macroadenoma. T1 postcontrast coronal and T2 coronal images: A1 tracts of anterior cerebral arteries (long black arrows) and vestigial tract of internal carotid artery (short black arrow) are encased by the tumor.

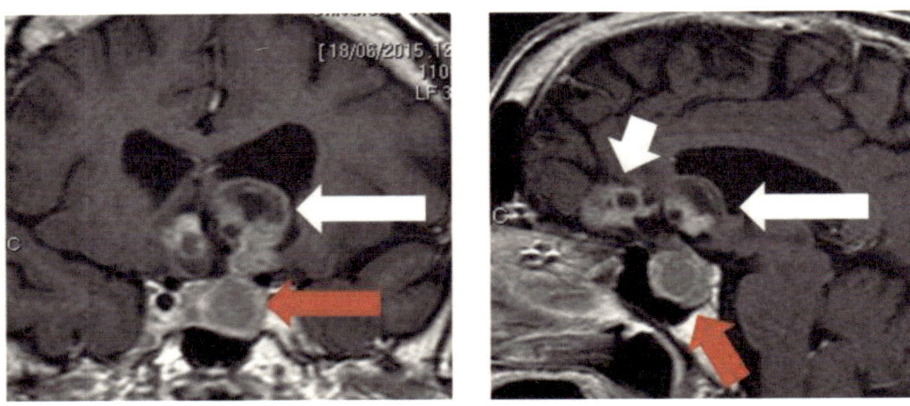

Figure 4. Invasive huge pituitary adenoma. T1 postcontrast coronal and sagittal images show intrasellar component of adenoma (red arrows), suprasellar diencephalic tumor component (long white arrows), and anterior frontal component of adenoma (short white arrow in sagittal slice).

were not above displaced (**Figures 3** and **4**): we programmed a staged transsphenoidal surgery, as other authors [4], programming the second stage when the tumor remnant would had been descended into the sellar cave. In order to perform the second programmed stage, neuronavigator was employed, as previously described, because anatomical landmarks could have become unclear because of the previous operation. For pituitary adenomas invading cavernous sinuses (**Figure 5**) and for tumors with anterior or lateral extension to frontal or temporal lobe (**Figure 4**), respectively, therapeutic strategy was to remove the median intrasuprasellar part of tumor, without performing access to cavernous sinus and without performing extensive transsphenoidal approach or transcranial approach to remove frontal and temporal tumor portions. Therapy for these tumoral portions was hypofractionated stereotactic radiotherapy (HSRT).

2.4. Surgery

Transsphenoidal surgery was performed through submucosal approach through one nostril, in 38 cases with the aid of angulated endoscope.

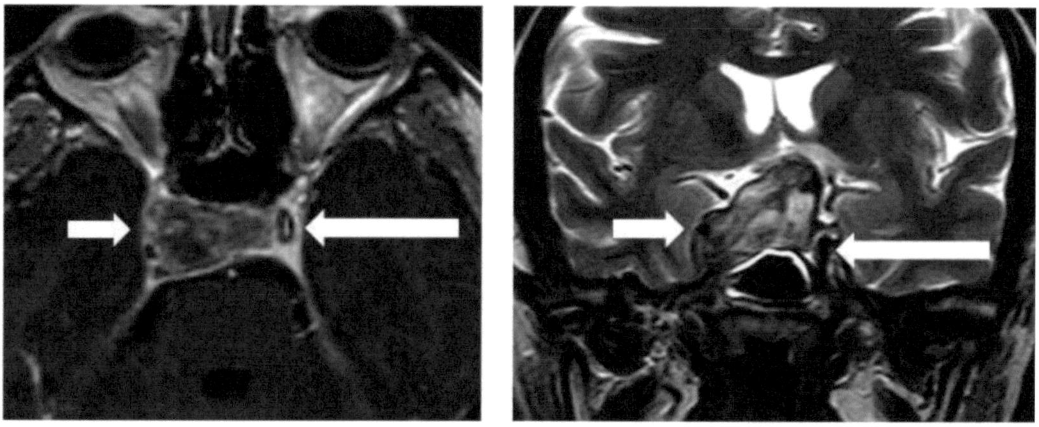

Figure 5. Hemorrhagic pituitary adenoma. T1 postcontrast Axial and T2 coronal image: invasion of right cavernous sinus (short black arrow) by adenoma is evident, while left cavernous sinus (long black arrow) is not invaded by the tumor.

The supine position [5] was used in all patients. In 71, the microsurgical approach was endoscope assisted. As previously described, in these voluminous tumors, if surgical removal starts from the central part of the adenoma, the suprasellar cisternal plane can precociously descend into the sella turcica, compressing portions of the tumor toward the lateral sides of the operative field (**Figure 6A**); therefore, these parts of tumor become difficult to remove, also with the aid of the endoscope. In this case, it is frequent damaging the suprasellar cisternal plane (intraoperative CSF leak) and the related possible complications as stretch of the optic chiasm and postoperative rhinoliquorrhea. The modified technique for these voluminous adenomas consisted in opening at the beginning only the lateral parts of peritumoral dura mater (**Figure 6B**). In this way, the central part of the dura mater remains in support of the central part of tumor and suprasellar cisternal plane. After removal of lateral parts of the tumor, the central part of peritumoral dura mater is opened and the central intrasellar and suprasellar parts of the tumor are removed [6].

Peritumoral anterior and/or posterior prepontine dura mater was infiltrated in all patients; surgical removal was conducted in each patient until the suprasellar arachnoidal plane, which was, at operative microscopic/endoscopic view, infiltrated by the tumor in 98 cases. Suprasellar arachnoidal plane was preserved in all patients but four, so that in these last patients, meticulous reconstruction of skull base defect was necessary to avoid postoperative rhinoliquorrhea. At operative view, the tumor in 39 patients invaded lateral sides of operative field that were medial wall of cavernous sinuses. Four patients were submitted, during an average period of 12 months, to two-staged transsphenoidal surgery; after first operation, because tumor remnant was voluminous and too close to optic chiasm, a second operation was performed after several months to achieve a satisfactory optic nerve decompression and possibility to perform a safe radiotherapic treatment. In one patient affected by macroadenoma with encasement of optic chiasm and A1 tracts of anterior cerebral arteries without displacement, the intrasellar and a quite small suprasellar portion of tumor were removed at surgery, and 6 months after surgery, the tumor remnant descended into the sellar cave.

Concerning the 12 and 5 patients presenting respectively temporal and frontal tumor extension, surgical strategy was to remove only the intrasellar and suprasellar median tumoral portion to decompress optic chiasm; MRI was performed after 1 month, and in no case, the

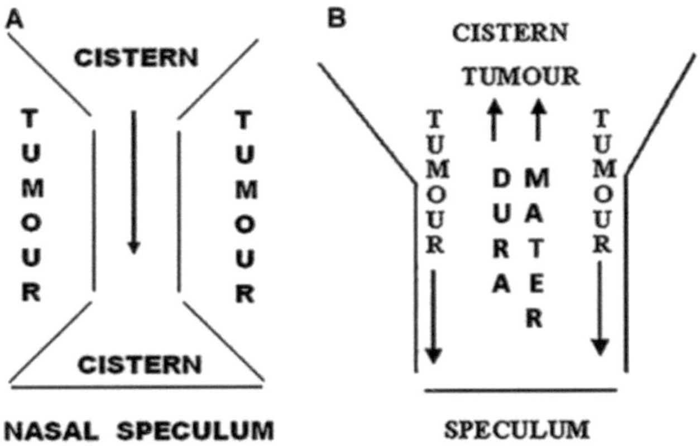

Figure 6. (A) Drawing of possible precocious intraoperative empty sella during inadequate transsphenoidal removal of huge pituitary adenomas: if tumor removal starts with the intrasellar and suprasellar central parts of the adenoma, the suprasellar cisternal plane can precociously go down into the sella turcica or even sphenoidal sinus, laterally compressing parts of the tumor, which should be difficult to be removed. (B) Drawing of the surgical technique. The lateral parts of the tumor are initially removed (long black arrows); the central part of the tumor at the beginning is left in situ in support of the cisternal plane.

lateral/frontal tumor remnant descended into the sella turcica. Hypofractionated radiotherapy was programmed also in these patients.

2.5. Postoperative radiotherapy

The treatment of choice for this series of patients was hypofractionated stereotactic radiotherapy (HSRT); the treatment was performed in all patients between 1 and 4 months after surgery. Only in one patient, radiotherapy was performed 5 years after surgery, although a clear initial regrowth had been documented after the second year of follow-up, but the patient during the years after surgery was controlled only by other specialists and the progressive tumor regrow was not well enlightened. HSRT was then performed when the tumor had become quite large and occupied the entire sellar cave but without suprasellar extension; patient preferred radiotherapy than a new operation. Radiotherapic centering was performed in all patients through 1.5 tesla MR images fused with CT images, and target was contoured on fused images. Relocatable stereotactic frame was employed for individuation of stereotactic coordinates; thermoplastic mask with byte was used to achieve the same head positioning at each fraction, but patient positioning was controlled through i-view system by radiographic anatomical landmarks. Organs at risk were contoured, and particular attention was paid to the dose adsorbed by optic chiasm, carotid arteries, intracavernous cranial nerves, diencephalus, and hippocampus. Radiotherapic dose administered was 40 Gy, delivered through 10 biweekly fractions. Concerning patients with suprasellar temporal and frontal tumor remnant, a complex radiotherapic treatment was planned and performed, delivering radiation dose both in the intrasellar operative field and at the anterior/lateral suprasellar tumor remnant, sparing in particular the optic chiasm between the two tumoral remnants, thanks to intensity-modulated radiotherapy (IMRT; **Figure 7**).

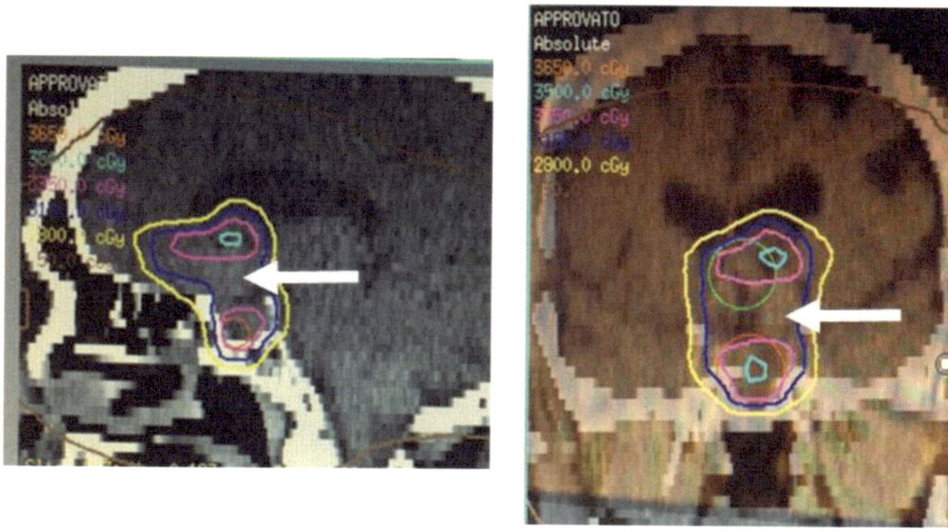

Figure 7. Complex radiotherapic treatment concerning case of **Figure 4**. Two targets were performed to treat intrasellar tumoral remnant and diencephalic tumor component, sparing neurovascular component.

Before radiotherapy, blood hormone dosages were assessed to test endocrinological status. Moreover, cognitive status was tested before and after radiotherapy once a year for the first 3 years and once at 2 years afterward, through neuropsychological test such as Mini-mental test, Rey-Osterrieth test (ROCF), Raven test, Stroop test, and verbal fluency test (COWAT).

Radiotherapic dose adsorbed by hippocampus was in all patients very low and however considerably less than the radiotherapic dose responsible of intellectual damages.

2.6. Results

In general, the modified technique allowed to achieve in our experience better results concerning intraoperative CSF leak (2.4% instead of 22.5%) and postoperative CSF fistula 0% instead of 7.4%), average time of postoperative stay in hospital (4.3 days instead of 8.2 days).

After surgery, all patients affected by visual acuity and campimetry impairment presented precocious improvement; out of the 16 patients affected by diplopia due to 3rd/4th/6th cranial nerve palsy, 14 patients presented total recovery during an average period of 4 weeks, one patient presented improvement and another remained unchanged. Postoperative hormonal status remained unchanged in all patients: neither improvement nor worsening than preoperative hormonal status occurred after surgery, and patients with preoperative hypopituitarism were submitted to hormonal substitutive therapy. Two patients presented rhinoliquorrhea after 2 and 5 weeks, respectively; they were treated by instillation of fibrin glue into the sphenoidal sinus under CT control [7].

One patient presented transitory sixth cranial nerve palsy with diplopia and complete recovery occurred after 2 months.

Concerning tumor removal, apparent total removal was performed in 51 patients, while in other 37, gross total removal was accomplished; tumor remnants located into the cavernous sinuses (45 cases), in frontal (5 cases), and temporal lobes (12 cases) were left in situ. During an average follow-up period of 9.7 years, after our protocol represented by conservative surgery followed by HSRT, only one patient presented a hemorrhagic tumor regrowth, 4 years after radiotherapy, with optic chiasm compression; transsphenoidal reoperation was performed and patient recovered visual deficit, and after 4 years from second surgery, no new tumor recurrence/regrow was registered. Leaving in situ small tumoral remnant adherent to suprasellar critical structures (diencephalus, A1 tracts of ACA), we often observed a progressive descent of tumoral remnant into the sellar cave (**Figure 8**), with possibility to perform a second transsphenoidal stage or radiotherapy.

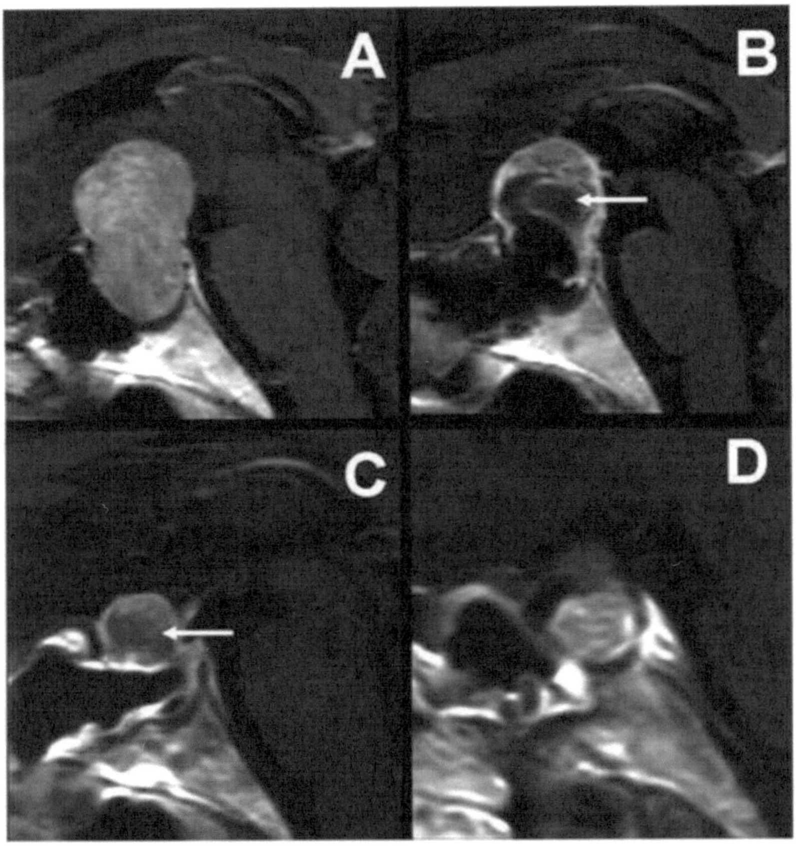

Figure 8. Case of huge pituitary adenoma with marked suprasellar extension operated on by transsphenoidal approach. In this case, a small suprasellar remnant was left in situ because it was very adherent to suprasellar structures. There was no occurrence of CSF leak during surgery, so that no particular material of apposition was put in the operative field, remaining free space under the suprasellar remnant. (A) Preoperative T1 sagittal postcontrast MRI. (B) Postoperative postcontrast MRI performed 5 days after surgery showing a small suprasellar remnant. It is noticeable a hypointensity area under the tumoral remnant (white arrow), representing free space under the tumoral remnant. (C) Postcontrast MRI performed 1 month after surgery; an initial descent of the tumoral remnant is evident and there is yet an area of hypointensity under the remnant itself (white arrow). (D) Postcontrast MRI performed 2 months after surgery: an ulterior descent into the sellar plane of the tumoral remnant is evident, with total decompression of suprasellar structures.

Concerning the 114 patients who presented preoperative hormonal deficit and therefore were under substitutive medical therapy, it should be noted that only in two of them, medical therapy with hydrocortisone was increased 6.4 and 8.1 years after HSRT; in the other, after an average follow-up period of 10.4 years, medical therapy remained unchanged, and quality of life was very satisfactory.

Regarding the 24 patients who were not affected by preoperative or postoperative hormonal deficit, in only one of them, replacement therapy with hydrocortisone and testosterone was necessary 6.7 years after HSRT. Three young female patients treated in our series 4, 6, and 7 years, respectively, after surgery and HSRT, experienced successful pregnancy.

Concerning neurocognitive status, no patient suffered from intellectual deterioration according to patients'/relatives' opinion and according to neurocognitive tests.

One patient presented rhinoliquorrhea after 2 months from radiotherapy, but he was treated conservatively with medical therapy (acetazolamide for 2 weeks), rest and life advices for 10 days with resolution.

No problems concerning trigemino-cardiac reflex [8, 9] were observed in this series.

2.7. Surgical findings vs. MR images

Concerning cavernous sinus invasion, intraoperative microsurgical/endoscopic view revealed a minor rate of cavernous sinus invasion than preoperative MR images. Moreover, operative view was the only possibility to detect dura mater infiltration and suprasellar arachnoidal infiltration by the tumor in many cases; this aspect was evident at preoperative MRI in those tumors which showed a clear invasive behavior (**Figure 4**). Intraoperative evidence of dura mater and suprasellar arachnoid infiltration significantly influenced our choice to perform postoperative hypofractionated radiotherapy.

2.8. Surgical removal of invasive pituitary adenomas

In consideration that pituitary adenomas are benign tumors, our first objective was to decompress neurological structures removing tumor as much as possible without causing new neurological deficit and without running high risks of life to remove small tumor remnants adherent to the suprasellar and laterosellar vital neurovascular structures. According to this objective, we did not perform tumor removal into the cavernous sinus and we did not perform any traction on the superior tumoral portion adherent to vital neurovascular structures (A1 tracts of anterior cerebral artery, diencephalus, optic chiasm), leaving in situ these small tumoral remnants. This conservative behavior allowed to achieve very satisfactory postoperative results in absence of neurological deficit; concerning tumoral remnant, postoperative MRI confirmed in all patients a progressive descent into the sellar cave of superior tumor remnants.

Our modified surgical technique is indicated for huge pituitary adenomas with marked suprasellar extension operated on by transsphenoidal surgery. The technique allows to prevent the occurrence of a precocious intraoperative descent of suprasellar cisternal plane and its related consequences above mentioned and to perform a tumor removal larger than patients operated with standard technique. When intraoperative CSF leak occurs, the surgeon has to fill the sphenoidal sinus and the sella turcica with material of apposition [10, 11], and this situation precludes, or however delays, the progressive descent into the sella turcica of the suprasellar tumoral remnant in case of gross total removal when the suprasellar tumoral remnant is adherent to suprasellar structures. Moreover, intraoperative CSF leak exposes patients to the risk of a postoperative rhinoliquorrea and its related eventual complications (cephalalgia, pneumoencephalus, subdural hematoma, and meningitis). On the contrary, when intraoperative CSF leak does not occur, an eventual tumoral remnant can descend into the sella turcica after few weeks (**Figure 8**) because of the absence of excessive presence of material of apposition.

2.9. Indication to postoperative radiotherapy and side effects

Nowadays, there is not yet a unique indication and modality to perform postoperative radiotherapy [12–14]. Some centers consider immediate postoperative radiation therapy in an attempt to prevent tumor regrowth, but risk of complications such as hypopituitarism, cerebrovascular disease, potential neurocognitive dysfunction, and a low long-term risk of secondary intracranial tumors are reported. Concerning these risks, it should be noted that they are usually related to conventional radiotherapy that was performed in the past decades, and a sufficiently long follow-up period is available. Concerning our experience with hypofractionated stereotactic radiotherapy, our data show that rate of side effects is extremely low, however considering that average follow-up period after HSRT is 9.8 years. No cerebrovascular disease, neurocognitive dysfunction, or secondary intracranial tumors were registered in our experience with HSRT. Concerning hypopituitarism, first of all, we have to consider that in the presented series, a relevant part of patients presented preoperative hypopituitarism; however, only three patients needed substitutive medical therapy (hydrocortisone and levothyroxine) respectively after 3, 5, and 6.4 years after radiotherapy. Finally, we registered that three young female patients treated in our series experienced successful pregnancy. Hypofractionated stereotactic radiotherapy was preferred to radiosurgery because the first one, in our experience, allowed a very satisfactory tumor control with negligible side effects; moreover, HSRT allows to treat also tumor remnants (**Figure 7**) more voluminous than radiosurgery, in absence of damages to the critical neurovascular structures of the pituitary-diencephalic region.

Finally, concerning timing of HSRT, in our patients, we performed the treatment as soon as the MRI showed the descent of the tumor remnant into the sellar cave (between 1 and 4 months); in the cases of tumor remnant into the cavernous sinuses, HSRT was performed between 1 and 2 months. Recurrence after radiotherapy occurred in the only patient who performed HSRT 5 years after surgery, when the tumor remnant had already regrown; it is known that effect of radiotherapy is better, as well as the tumor remnant is small. Therefore, our indication is that HSRT in voluminous invasive pituitary adenomas should be performed as soon as possible, but ideally when tumor remnant has been descended into the sellar cave and optic chiasm has been decompressed.

One important aspect is the correct evaluation of postoperative MRIs after transsphenoidal surgery for huge pituitary adenomas; usually, the neurosurgeon evaluates by himself the extent of removal, and usually, MRI is significant 2–3 months after surgery. Precocious MRIs within the 2–4 weeks after surgery are not so significant for evaluation of tumor removal, because of the presence of material of apposition, because of the absence of tumor capsule collapse, etc. (**Figures 9–11**).

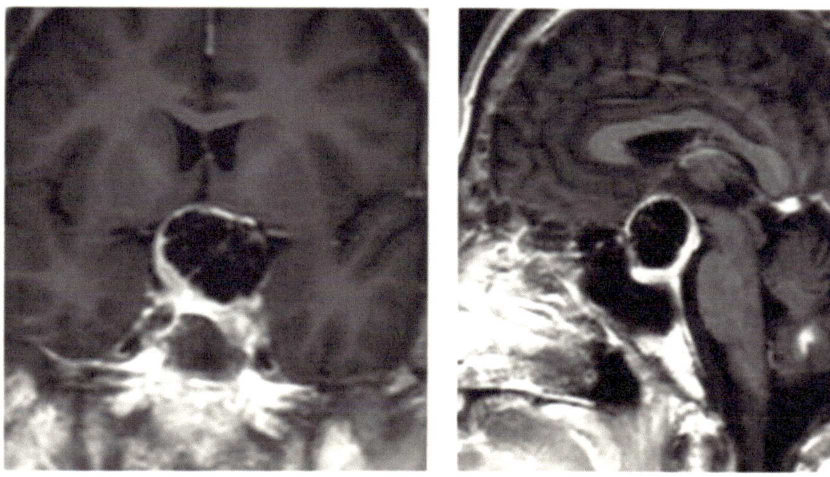

Figure 9. Preoperative MRI of hemorrhagic huge pituitary adenoma. Optic chiasm, pituitary stalk, and chiasmatic arachnoid cistern are not evident because of tumor compression.

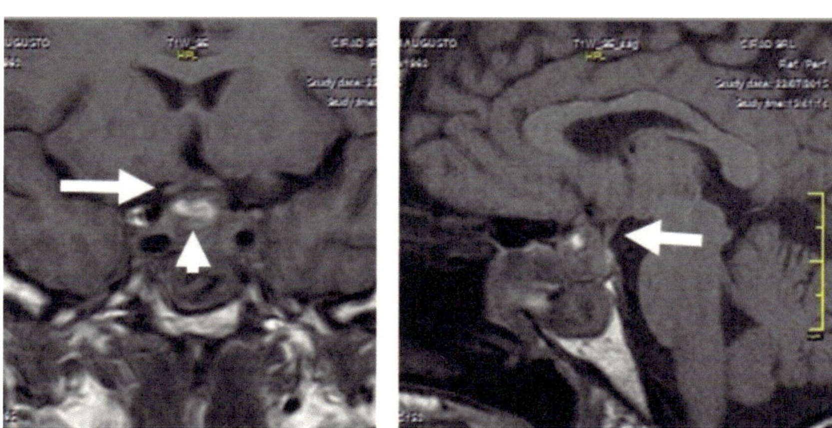

Figure 10. Precocious postoperative MRI performed 7 days after surgery. Coronal image: optic chiasm is now evident (white arrow); a slight hyperintense signal is evident (white arrow head), corresponding to hemostatic material. Sagittal image: pituitary stalk is now evident.

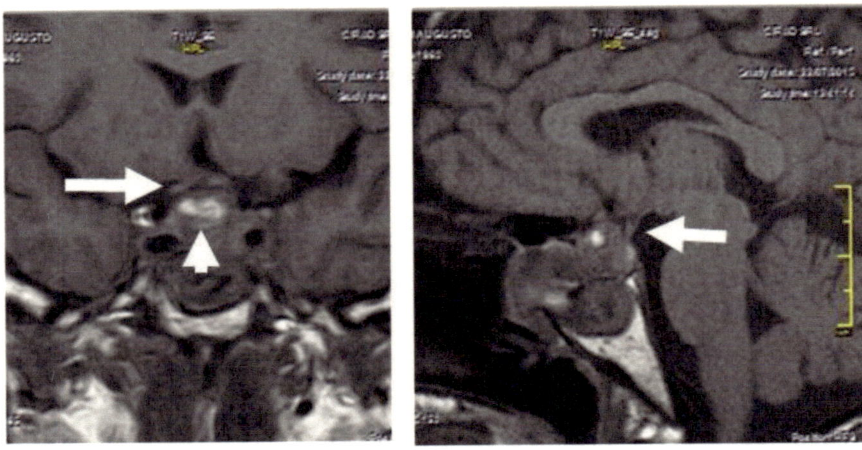

Figure 11. Postoperative MRI performed 2 months after surgery showing an optimal decompression of suprasellar structures. Coronal image: optic chiasm (long white arrow), pituitary stalk (white arrow head), and chiasmatic cistern (short white arrow) are evident and are now well visible compared to precocious postoperative MRI. Sagittal image: chiasmatic cistern is well visible (white arrow).

3. Conclusions

In our experience, the presented modified transsphenoidal microsurgical technique for removal of huge pituitary adenomas with marked suprasellar extension minimizes damages to the suprasellar cisternal plane, and therefore, intraoperative CSF leak is very rare; total removal can be achieved with higher percentage rate than patients operated with standard technique however in noninvasive adenomas. Postoperative stay in hospital is shorter, and nasal packing can be removed in the first postoperative day. For huge invasive dumbbell-shaped adenomas, personalized treatment should be performed according to the degree of neurovascular structures encasement (optic chiasm, diencephalus, cavernous sinuses, and A1 tracts of anterior cerebral arteries).

Author details

Mario Francesco Fraioli[1]*, Andrea Pagano[1], Bernardo Fraioli[2] and Pierpaolo Lunardi[1]

*Address all correspondence to: mff77@libero.it

1 Department of Neurosurgery, University of Rome Tor Vergata, Roma, Italy

2 Department of Radiotherapy and Radiosurgery, CIRAD Villa Benedetta, Roma, Italy

References

[1] Couldwell WT. Transsphenoidal and transcranial surgery for pituitary adenomas. Journal of Neuro-Oncology. 2004;**69**(1-3):237-256

[2] Youssef AS, Agazzi S, van Loveren HR. Transcranial surgery for pituitary adenomas. Neurosurgery. 2005;**57**(1 Suppl):168-175

[3] Fraioli B, Esposito V, Liccardo G, Giuffrè R, Cantore G. The supine position for transsphenoidal surgery. Neurosurgical Review. 1994;**17**(4):275-276

[4] Fraioli MF, Catena E, Lecce M, Fraioli B. Transsphenoidal removal of huge pituitary adenomas with marked suprasellar extension: Results with modified surgical technique. Clinical Neurology and Neurosurgery. Apr 2013;**115**(4):450-453. DOI: 10.1016/j.clineuro.2012.06.019 [Epub Jul 7, 2012]

[5] Fraioli B, Pastore FS, Floris R, Vagnozzi R, Simonetti G, Liccardo G, et al. Computed tomography-guided transsphenoidal closure of postsurgical cerebrospinal fluid fistula: A transmucosal needle technique. Surgical Neurology. 1997;**48**(4):409-413

[6] Kaptain GJ, Kanter AS, Hamilton DK, Laws ER. Management and implications of intraoperative cerebrospinal fluid leak in transnasoseptal transsphenoidal microsurgery. Neurosurgery. 2011;**68**(1 Suppl. Operative):144-151

[7] Dusick JR, Mattozo CA, Esposito F, Kelly DF. Bio glue for prevention of post-operative cerebrospinal fluid leaks in transsphenoidal surgery: Acaseseries. Surgical Neurology. 2006;**66**(4):371-376

[8] Takakura K, Teramoto A. Management of huge pituitary adenomas. Acta Neurochirurgica Supplement. 1996;**65**:13-15

[9] Colin P, Jovenin N, Delemer B, Caron J, Grulet H, Hecart AC, et al. Treatment of pituitary adenomas by fractionated stereotactic radiotherapy: A prospective study of 110 patients. International Journal of Radiation Oncology, Biology, Physics. 2005;**62**: 333-341

[10] Fahlbusch R, Honegger J, Paulus W, Huk W, Buchfelder M. Surgical treatment of cranio: Experience with 168 patients. Journal of Neurosurgery. 1999;**90**(2):237-250

[11] Schaller B. Trigemino-cardiac reflex during transsphenoidal surgery for pituitary adenomas. Clinical Neurology and Neurosurgery. 2005;**107**(6):468-474

[12] Schaller BJ, Filis A, Buchfelder M. Trigemino-cardiacreflex in humans initiated by peripheral stimulation during neurosurgical skull-base operations. Its first description. Acta Neurochirurgica. 2008;**150**(7):715-718

[13] Giaj Levra N, Sicignano G, Fiorentino A, Fersino S, Ricchetti F, Mazzola R, Naccarato S, Ruggieri R, Alongi F. Whole brain radiotherapy with hippocampal avoidance and simultaneous integrated boost for brain metastases: A dosimetric volumetric-modulated arc therapy study. La Radiologia Medica. Jan 2016;**121**(1):60-69. DOI: 10.1007/s11547-015-0563-8 [Epub Aug 1, 2015]

[14] Greene-Schloesser D, Robbins ME. Radiation-induced cognitive impairment-from bench to bedside. Neuro-Oncology. Sep 2012;**14**(Suppl 4):iv37-iv44. DOI: 10.1093/neuonc/nos196 (Review)

Chapter 3

Transoral Robotic Surgery Applied to the Skull Base

Dorian Chauvet and Stephane Hans

Additional information is available at the end of the chapter

http://dx.doi.org/10.5772/intechopen.81048

Abstract

Skull base surgery has been developed with transsphenoidal approaches to reach the sella and especially the pituitary tumors. Transnasal endoscopic technique has become the gold standard for many years. Indeed, the intraoperative view with specific endoscope is very good, and thus the gross total of pituitary adenomas removal rates have been increased. Nevertheless, why has not this technique been challenged, especially given the potential rhinologic side effects and 2D vision? Robotic surgery with the da Vinci system is now well known all over the world. Transoral robotic surgery (TORS) is also commonly used in head and neck cancer with satisfying results. In this ENT approach, the da Vinci videoendoscope looks downward; we had the idea to place it behind the hard palate in order to look upward. Therefore, from cadaveric studies to clinical "première mondiale," we developed an innovative TORS to reach the sella and to remove pituitary tumors.

Keywords: transoral robotic surgery, pituitary adenoma, da Vinci system, skull base surgery, robot-assisted surgery, transsphenoidal surgery

1. Introduction

Initial attempts at transsphenoidal surgery were first tested at the beginning of the twentieth century by early neurosurgeons [1]. Over the past 30 years, endoscopic transnasal techniques have become the gold standard, avoiding scares and allowing a better field of vision into the nasal narrow corridor. However, endoscopic approaches continue to present several inconveniences such as the narrowness of the operative corridor, the potential rhinologic side effects after removal of endonasal structures (such as turbinates or nasal septum), the two-dimensional vision, and a quite long learning curve. One could also mention the ergonomic discomfort for the surgeon to perform fine dissection requiring two hands compared to microscopic classic dissection.

For many years, robotic surgery with the da Vinci system (Intuitive Surgical Inc., Sunnyvale, CA, USA) has been increasingly adopted, especially in urology [2] and gynecology [3]. This system offers increased freedom of movement within narrow corridors, three-dimensional visualization, motion scaling, and tremor filtration [4]. Moreover, the ergonomic comfort for the surgeon has improved. Recently, robot-assisted surgery has been performed for pharyngeal and laryngeal cancers in a minimally invasive perspective [5–7], leading to a new concept of *transoral robotic surgery* (TORS).

Concerning the neurosurgical field and especially the skull base field, literature with da Vinci surgery remains very poor, including a few cadaveric odontoidectomies [8–10] and one case report [11]. Moreover, it has to be mentioned that robotic supratentorial approaches by keyhole craniotomies have failed on cadavers [12].

In 1985, Crockard wrote that "the transoral surgical approach allows access to structures from the sphenoid sinus rostrally to the fourth cervical vertebral body caudally" [13]. Despite this pioneer reference and the new technical opportunities given by robot-assisted surgery, no TORS has been attempted to reach the sella turcica. Thus, we developed an innovative TORS for skull base in three steps: cadaveric study [14], anatomical general work [15], and clinical proof of concept [16].

2. Cadaveric study

2.1. Methods

Dissections were performed at the "Ecole Européenne de Chirurgie" with the da Vinci S HD 4 arms system. Regarding the anatomical consideration, only three arms were used (videoendoscope arm and two instrument arms). The system stood at the head of the cadaver, placed supine next to a C-arm fluoroscope (operative room plan in **Figure 1**).

A mouth retractor (type Doyen, Landanger®) was placed to get the usual transoral exposition. The soft palate was retracted using two rubber catheters introduced into the nose and pulled out by the mouth. Additionally, the tongue could be retracted with a stitch as well. An 8.5-mm 30° angled binocular endoscope, a 5-mm EndoWrist® Maryland dissector articulated, and a 5-mm EndoWrist® Monopolar cautery instrument were attached on the patient cart, respectively, on the middle, right, and left arms of the system. The three arms were brought into the oral cavity: the 30° videoendoscope arm facing upward on the midline and the two other robotic arms laterally, respecting teeth and labial commissures of the mouth (see **Figure 2**).

It is mandatory to mention that two surgeons were necessary to perform the dissection: one author, head and neck surgeon (SH), at the console and the other one, neurosurgeon (DC), at the bedside. The latter was necessary to perform suction and to prevent a robotic arm conflict with the oral cavity structures during the mucosal dissection. Afterward, the second surgeon performed the bone drilling and the sellar opening. Four phases can be defined:

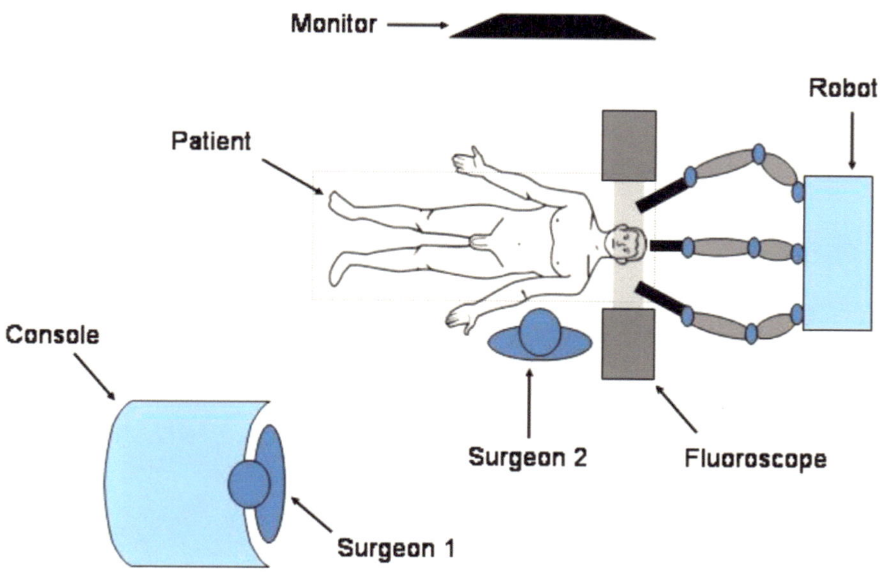

Figure 1. Schematic view of the operating room. Surgeon 1 is the head and neck surgeon working at the console (SH) and Surgeon 2 is the neurosurgeon working at the bedside (DC) [14].

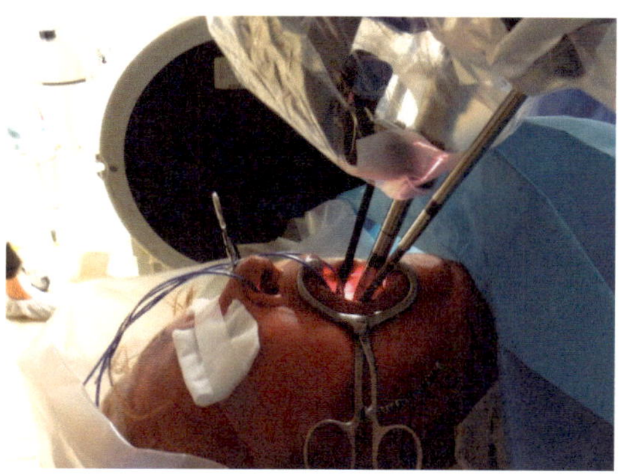

Figure 2. Lateral intraoperative view. The three robotic arms stand in the oral cavity that is open with a mouth retractor. The retraction of the soft palate is performed using two rubber catheters introduced in the nose and pulled out by the mouth. In the background, the C-arm fluoroscope for intraoperative 2D lateral control [14].

2.1.1. Mucosal time

Once the endoscope was pushed beyond the hard palate, an upward view of the cavum and the choanae was obtained. The surgeon at the console performed the flap of the posterior cavum mucosa, which corresponded to the mucosa covering anteriorly and inferiorly the sphenoidal rostrum (see **Figure 3**).

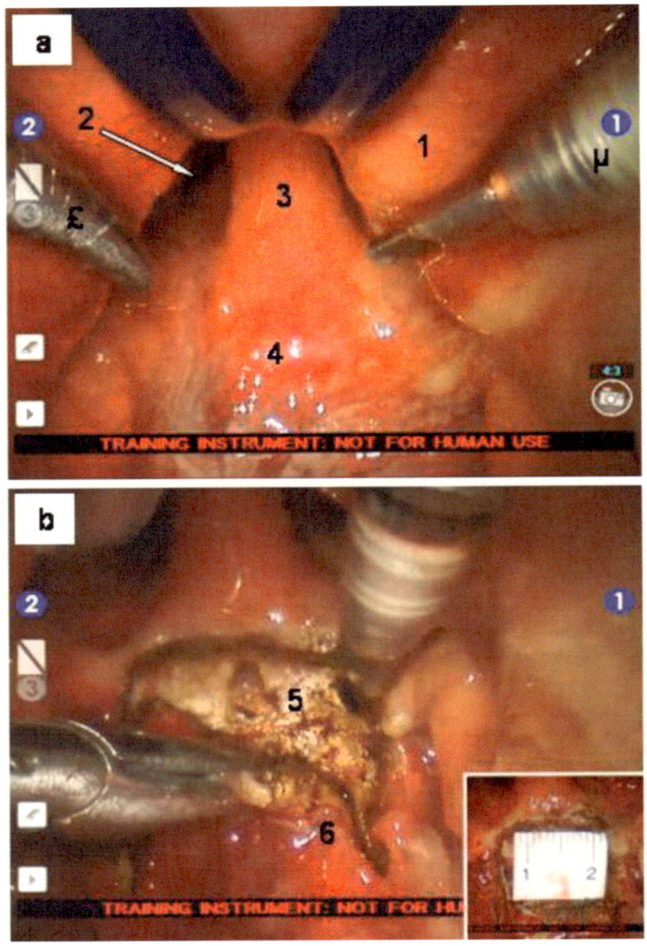

Figure 3. Intraoperative view with the 30° endoscope within the cavum. (a) The soft palate (1) is retracted using two rubber catheters at the top of the picture. The choanae are well visualized (right choana) (2). (3) indicates a decisive landmark that corresponds to the articulation between the vomer and the sphenoid. (4) is the mucosa of the cavum and (μ) and (£) are monopolar cautery and Maryland dissector, respectively. (b) The mucosal flap (6) is dissected with a caudal base in order to discover a key point that corresponds to the junction between the alea of the vomer (5) and the sphenoid itself; the picture on the right bottom corner indicates the size of the flap, approximately 15 mm width [14].

2.1.2. *Sphenoid time*

Afterward, the surgeons' roles changed, and the left robotic arm was removed to provide space to the neurosurgeon at the bedside. As the da Vinci system has no bony instruments, the opening of the sphenoid sinus was performed by the neurosurgeon, watching his progression on the 2D flat-panel screen. The first surgeon sitting at the console offered a supplementary intraoperative control with 3D view and could perform suction thanks to a dedicated robotic tool—8 mm EndoWrist® One™ suction irrigator. An electric motor (Bien-Air®) was employed with matchstick burs attached on a slightly angled handpiece. Another drilling system was employed in the clinical study (see below) [16]. Before drilling the sphenoid, the attack angle of the drill was verified by a lateral fluoroscopy. The sphenoid sinus was opened and enlarged with kerrison punch to get a wide vision of the sella turcica (see **Figure 4**).

2.1.3. Sellar time

The sellar floor was opened with the drill and the kerrison punch. The robotic arms were inserted into the sphenoid sinus deeply to appreciate the maneuverability of the da Vinci EndoWrist® instruments in such a narrow space. The dura mater opened the robotic monopolar cautery. In clinical study [16], other instruments were used to open the dura (see below). The pituitary gland resection of the cadavers was attempted, and anatomical suprasellar structures were identified (see **Figure 5**).

2.1.4. Closure

Suture of the flap was attempted.

Times of each step were assessed and unexpected difficulties were reported.

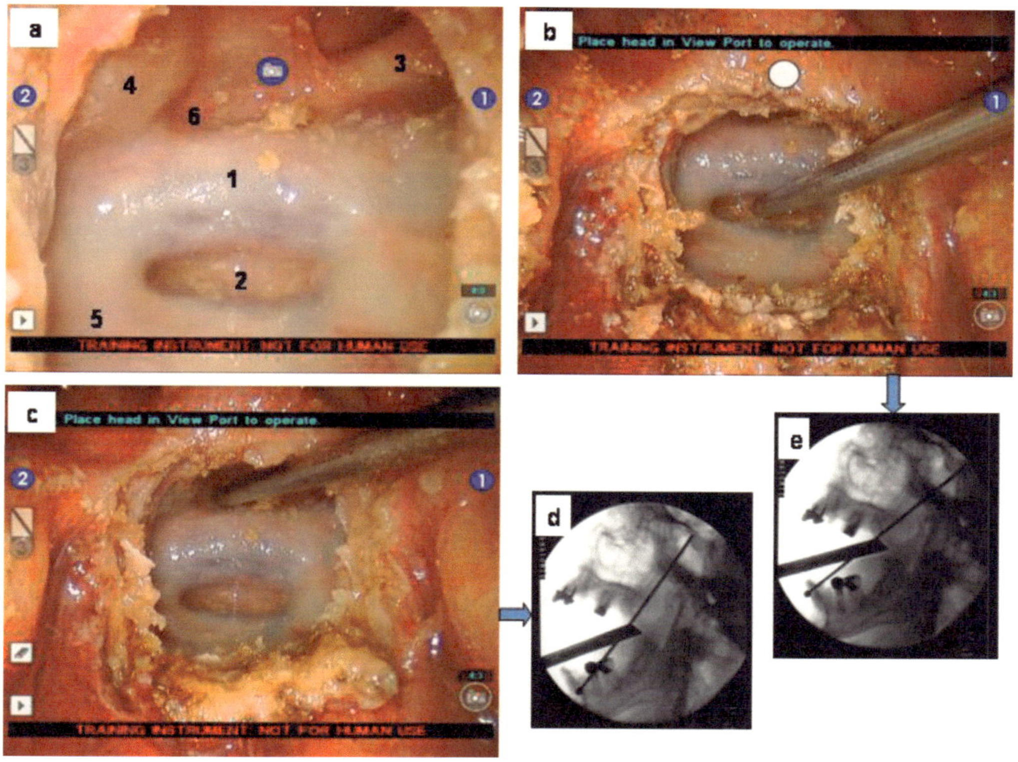

Figure 4. Intraoperative endoscopic view of the sella turcica. (a) Anatomical structures of the sphenoid sinus: (1) sellar floor, (2) dorsum sellae that is well pneumatized, (3) left optic nerve protuberance, (4) right carotid protuberance—sellar portion, (5) right carotid protuberance—clival portion, and (6) opto-carotid recess. (b) Dissector placed in the pneumatized dorsum sellae and the corresponding fluoroscopic lateral picture (e). (c) Dissector inserted in front of the anterior wall of the sella and the corresponding fluoroscopic view (d) [14].

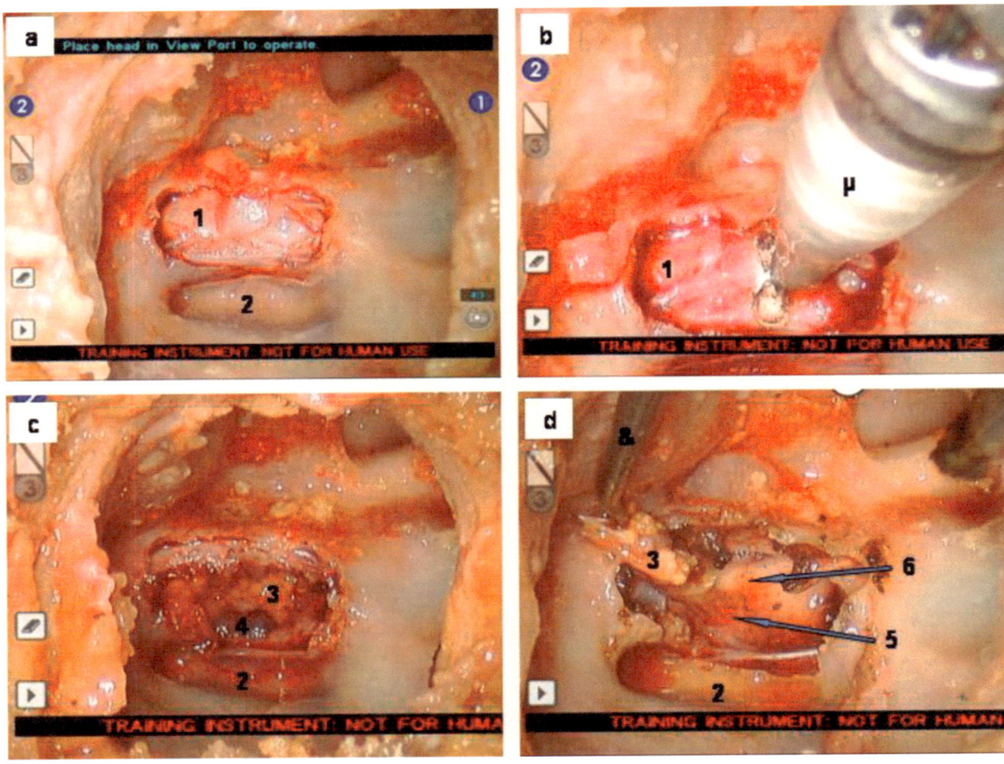

Figure 5. Intraoperative view of the pituitary fossa dissection. (a) View after sellar floor removal. (b) Cauterization of the sellar dura with the monopolar cautery (μ). (c) View during pituitary gland resection. (d) Final view after removal. Legends: (1) sellar dura, (2) pneumatized dorsum sellae, (3) pituitary gland, (4) sellar diaphragm, (5) pituitary stalk retracted by a hook (6), and (7) optic chiasm [14].

2.2. Results

A total of 11 cadavers were dissected. Despite the anatomical heterogeneities of the specimens, the setup was easy, and the visualization of the cavum was large with a perfect view. At that time, two structures were required as reference points: both sides of choana and the posterior border of the vomer that provided an accurate midline landmark. As in other transsphenoidal approaches, keeping the dissection on the midline was mandatory. We did not experience lateral deviation in our dissections. The cavum mucosa was not always dissected in a whole flap (n = 5) as tissues of cadavers were sometimes fragile. All of the soft tissue sequence was performed easily with enough space to use the robotic instruments and without any tension on the oral cavity structures, especially the soft palate. Once the mucosal flap was raised, we defined a key point to enter the sphenoid sinus, which corresponded to the junction between the vomer and the sphenoid itself (see **Figure 3**).

All sphenoidal sinuses were "sellar," which meant that the pneumatization was posterior to the anterior wall of the sella turcica. The bony sequence was achieved by placing the motor handpiece in the right labial commissure of the mouth. Indeed, the lateral movement of the handpiece, following naturally the lower teeth curve from the midline to the labial commissure, allowed an opening of the angle of work to the skull base (see **Figure 6**). The latter was defined by the angle between the horizontal line passing through the hard palate and the projected line of the drill (as seen in **Figure 6** by dotted lines), which was placed at the midline and then in the labial commissure. From these comparative cadavers' measurements, we observed that the mean angles of work were 55° (min 48, max 62) and 71.5° (min 67, max 76) for the midline and the lateral positions, respectively. Thus, we hypothesized that the mean angle of work gain placing the drill in the labial commissure was +16.5°.

In all dissections, this procedure had succeeded in approaching the sella turcica, and we had encountered no difficulty in our approach. To prevent a lateral deviation of the drilling, the angled feature of the handpiece was decisive. Opening the sphenoid sinus was achieved quickly (approximately 10 min), depending on the thickness of the sphenoidal rostrum. The videoendoscope was successfully introduced in this sinus during all dissections and thus had provided a wide 3D view of the sella turcica and its surrounding structures (as shown in **Figure 5**). Then, the pituitary fossa was opened with a thinner diamond drill. The robotic arms reached the sella turcica in all procedures with a correct manageability. The normal pituitary gland was removed with robotic instruments (see **Figure 7**). The final view of the pituitary stalk and the optic chiasm was obtained. Closure attempts to suture the dura were impossible, and it was quite difficult to suture the flap due to the fragile mucosa. At the end of the dissection, inspection of the oral cavity revealed no injury. The mean robotic setup time was 20 minutes (range, 10–35 minutes); the mean mucosal time was 10 minutes (range, 5–15 minutes); and the combined sphenoid and sellar time was 30 minutes (range, 15–60 minutes).

In conclusion these cadaveric preliminary results were very promising and TORS skull base seemed reproducible, awaiting further clinical trial.

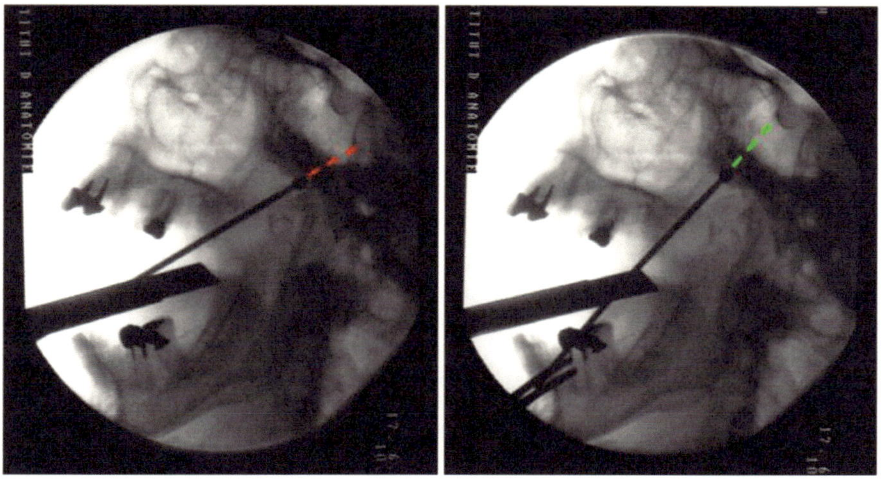

Figure 6. Fluoroscopic lateral views, the endoscope standing at the midline of the mouth. On the left, the matchstick drill is inserted at the midline, and its projection on the sphenoid bone virtually meets the clivus (red-dotted line). On the contrary on the right picture, the bur is placed in the labial commissure, and its projection clearly meets the sella turcica (green-dotted line). This shows how the angle of work to the skull base is increased when the instruments are placed laterally in the oral cavity [14].

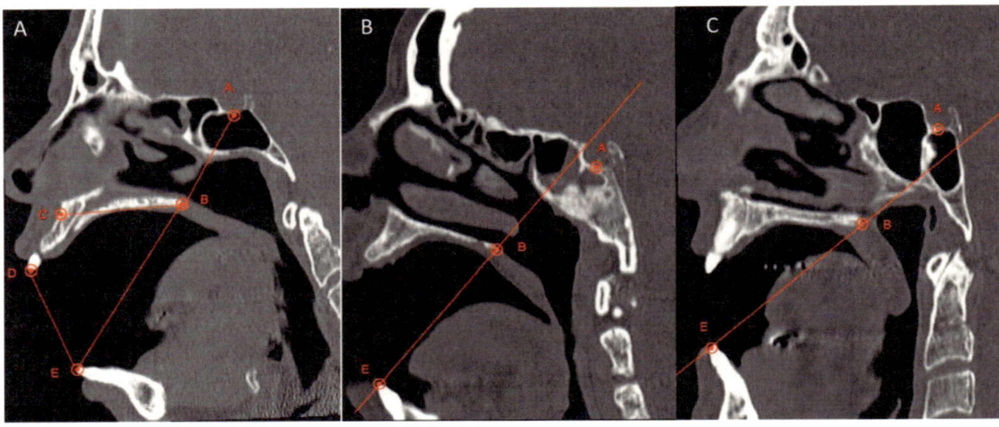

Figure 7. CT scan bony window sagittal midline views. (A) Description of the different points: A, sella turcica point; B, posterior palatine point; C, anterior palatine point; D, maxillary dental point; and E, mandibular point. Notice that the (BE) line is projected on point A on this picture. (B) Presellar projection of (BE) line. (C) Postsellar projection of (BE) line [15].

3. Anatomical study

3.1. Methods

This prospective single-center study hypothesized that TORS for skull base would be feasible in the majority of patients, regardless of their anatomical features [15]. Thus, we studied some anatomical criteria on radiological data from patients requiring a cerebral CT scan for neurological issues. Patients were asked to open their mouth as large as they could during the CT scan, without any retractor. Patients with a history of endonasal surgery, sinus disease, and/or skull base pathology were excluded. After imaging acquisition, we also excluded patients with mouth opening inferior to 30 mm, as this threshold distance was far from the value with the usual mouth retractor [14]. CT scans were performed on a Somatom 16, Siemens. A double lecture was performed by one neurosurgeon and one neuroradiologist, who both collected the following data.

Firstly, on a sagittal midline view, we defined five points for each patients corresponding with strategic landmarks (see **Figure 7**), such as:

- Point A: the lowest point of the sella turcica.
- Point B: the most posterior palatine bone point.
- Point C: the most anterior palatine bone point.
- Point D: the maxillary dental point, at the tip of superior incisor.
- Point E: the mandibular dental point, at the tip of inferior incisor.

CT measurements also included four distances between the previous points, such as:

- [DE] for mouth opening
- [BC] for the length of the palate
- [AB] for the distance between the posterior edge of the palate and the sella
- [BE] for the distance between inferior incisors and posterior edge of the palate

Then, we examined from these landmarks the projection of the dental palatine line (aka (BE) line) on the sella. Patients were classified in three categories: projection anterior to point A of the sella (aka presellar projection), on point A, and posterior to point A (aka postsellar projection) (see **Figure 7A–C**, respectively). Finally, the alpha angle, named α, was determined as the angle between the horizontal palatine (BC) line and the dental palatine (BE) line (see **Figure 8A** and **B**).

Secondly, a 25° rotation from point B was made on the axial view to obtain a parasagittal oblique view (see **Figure 8C** and **D**) that corresponded to a specific intraoperative plane (see **Figure 8E**). Indeed, this virtual plane included the intraoperative surgical position of the robotic instruments, as surgical tools are placed at the labial commissures of the mouth. On this oblique view, point B was the same posterior palatine point, but the points C, E, and A changed into C′, E′, and A′, respectively, the parasagittal anterior palatine point, the parasagittal mandibular point, and the parasagittal lowest sella turcica point (see **Figure 8D**). The (BE′) line was projected on the sella turcica, and we determined whether it was presellar, postsellar, or on point A′ of the sella. Moreover, the α′ angle was the angle between the BE′ and BC′ lines. A comparison of α and α′ angle was performed. Thus, we were able to virtually compare if a lateral access changed the sella exposure.

Finally, pneumatization of the sphenoid sinus was defined according to the three physiological states that are concha, presellar, and sellar sphenoid sinus [17].

As a factor of surgical feasibility, we chose the projection of the dental palatine (BE) line on the sella. Thus, we separated the patients into two groups: the "straight approach" group with a presellar projection and the "no straight approach" group (with projection on point A of the sella and postsellar projection). Our statistical analysis included the following tests: the Kolmogorov-Smirnov normality test, the F-test for equality of variances, and the Student's t-test for patients' characteristics and comparison according to straight approach.

3.2. Results

A total of 38 cerebral CT scans were performed; out of those, 30 exams were assessed (mean patients' age = 57 years old); 8 patients were excluded because their mouth aperture was inferior to 30 mm. For all patients, the average mouth opening, aka [DE], was 39.4 mm IC 95% [36–42.8] and the length of the palate, aka [BC], was 47.4 mm IC 95% [45.2–49.5]. The distance between the inferior incisors and posterior edge of the hard palate, aka [BE], was measured at 69.5 mm IC 95% [67–72]. The average distance between the posterior edge of the palate

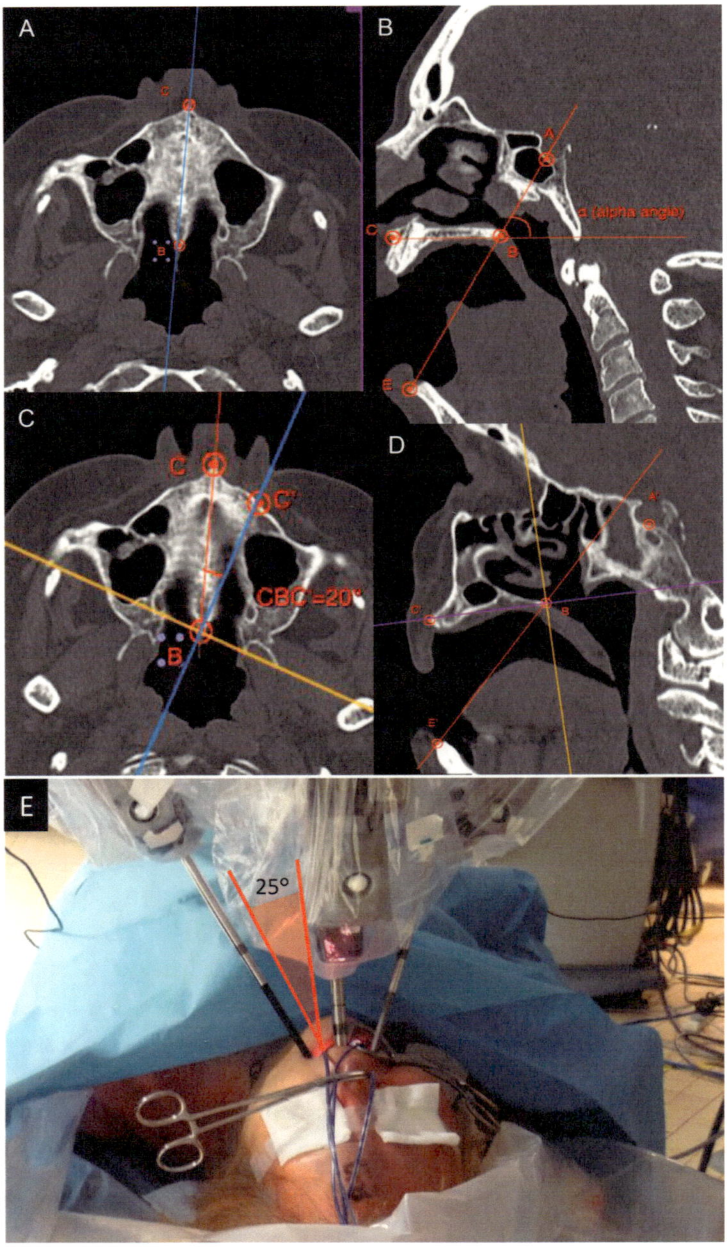

Figure 8. (A and B) Sagittal projections on midline: axial projection of the anterior maxillary point (point C) and the posterior palatine point (point B) and the midline sagittal view, the α (alpha angle) on the midline, determined as the angle between the BE line and the BC line. (C) and (D) Sagittal projections with lateral rotation of 25°. Axis rotation defined a parasagittal anterior maxillary point (point C′) and the parasagittal view with the parasagittal mandibular point (point E′) and the parasagittal sella turcica point (point A′). The posterior palatine point is fixed. (E) Photograph from cadaveric dissection of TORS at the bedside of the cadaver. The robotic instruments are placed into the oral cavity with a 25° angle (represented with a red triangle) between the endoscope at the midline and the dissector laterally [15].

[DE] mouth opening value (mm)	Sensitivity (%)	Specificity (%)
36.0	100.0	58.3
38.7	83.3	58.3
38.9	**83.3**	**70.8**
39.4	66.7	75.0
43.2	66.6	83.3
44.8	50.0	87.5
52.6	16.6	100.0

Table 1. Sensibility and specificity of mouth opening [DE] to predict the straight approach feasibility [15].

and the sella, aka [AB], was 43.1 mm IC 95% [41.5–44.7]. In our series, 2 patients (6%) had a presellar sinus and 28 patients (94%) had a sellar sphenoid sinus; we did not find any patient with concha sphenoid sinus.

Concerning our study of (BE) line projections on the sella, we described some dramatic changes between the midline plane and oblique plane. We found that 40% of patients ($n = 12$) had a (BE) line projection that moved forward when studied in the oblique plane, from the projection on A point to the presellar projection. Additionally, both angles, alpha α and α', were significantly different ($p < 0.05$), respectively, 59.3° IC 95% [56.1–62.4] and 64.7° IC 95% [62.1–67.3]. It tends to show that the axis of the instruments at the labial commissure of the mouth opened the working angle to the skull base.

Regarding our straight approach feasibility hypothesis, the only significant predictive factor was the spontaneous mouth opening [DE] ($p < 0.05$). We also observed that a mouth opening of 38.9 mm is sufficient to obtain a sensitivity of 83% and a specificity of 70.8% to predict our straight approach hypothesis (see **Table 1**).

Consequently, these data emphasized that the physiological maximal mouth opening could be an excellent predictive factor for feasibility of TORS. However, it seemed obvious that patients suffering from trismus could not be included in the further clinical study.

4. Clinical study

4.1. Methods

This prospective clinical study confirms the accessibility of the sella with TORS. It was conducted after validation of the French ethic committee and registration in Clinical Trials NCT02743442. The patients were referred to our institution, Rothschild Foundation, Paris, after the discovery of the sellar tumor, mostly revealed by visual symptoms. Once prolactinoma was excluded, surgical removal was decided, and the patient was informed of dedicated potential TORS risks (mastication difficulties, temporomandibular pain, hypernasal speech, and sore throat). A preoperative "open mouth" skull base CT scan was performed to envision the accessibility of the sella, as previously described [15]. The setup of the OR was the same than in our cadaveric study (see **Figure 1**). The only difference was that we used a da Vinci SI HD 4 arms system (Intuitive Surgical®, Sunnyvale, CA, USA). A general anesthesia was performed with the intubation placed on the left labial commissure.

The four surgical phases were the same as described above in the cadaveric work, except that a few modifications are described in the following lines.

4.1.1. Mucosal time

Mucosa of the posterior cavum was dissected into a "U-shaped" flap, instead of a caudal base flap (as in **Figure 3**), because we anticipated the possibility to raise the flap into the sella in case of CSF leak. During the next phases, this flap was positioned in the right choanae to facilitate sphenoidal approach.

4.1.2. Sphenoid time

The drilling of the key point was performed with a Midas Rex® Legend Stylus®, which offered an angled handpiece. Moreover, we used some diamond matchstick burs.

4.1.3. Sellar time and adenoma removal

For the dural opening, we prefer a CO_2 flexible Laser (Luminis®) guided by the robotic instruments rather than the monopolar cautery of the system. We must remind the reader that the da Vinci system has no dedicated instruments for pituitary surgery, so that the tumor removal was performed with curettes by the neurosurgeon at the patient's side (see **Figure 9**).

4.1.4. Closure

After removal, oxidized regenerated cellulose was placed against the sellar wall, and the mucosal flap was reapplied and sometimes glued. We did not try to suture the flap in the clinical trial, because preliminary works were mitigated.

Outcome measures included several criteria, such as preoperative data (i.e., visual function, radiological features of the tumor, open mouth CT scan data), intraoperative observations (i.e., exposure quality on the cavum and the sella, CSF leak occurrence, operative time for each phase, mucosal lesions in the oral cavity at the end of the procedure), and postoperative data. The latter were divided into two categories: TORS side effects (mastication dysfunction, temporomandibular pain, hypernasal speech, sore throat) and usual pituitary adenoma surgery outcomes/complications (vision status, CSF leak, meningitis, diabetes insipidus, hypopituitarism).

4.2. Results

Preoperative clinical data: a total of seven patients were included (five females, two males; mean age 46 years old). All presented with visual disturbance explained by bitemporal hemianopsia, except one patient who was operated on regarding the growth of his sellar tumor.

http://dx.doi.org/10.5772/intechopen.81048

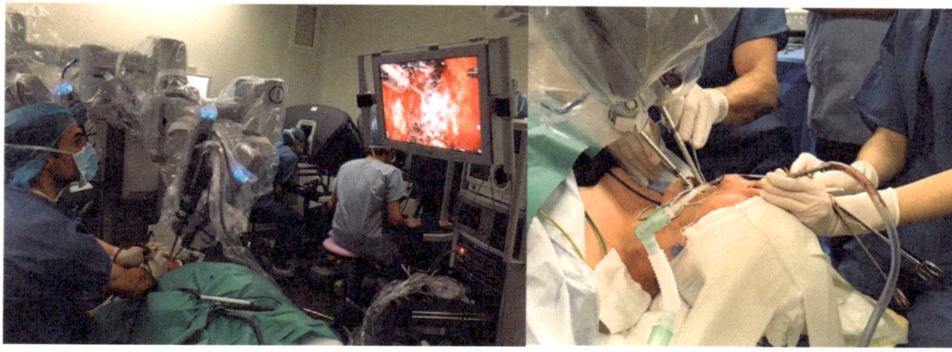

Figure 9. Operative views during the sphenoid and sellar times. The neurosurgeon (DC) performs the drilling at the bedside with his two hands placed at the labial commissure. An additional suction can be placed in the nasal cavity [16].

Preoperative radiological data: concerning radiological findings, five tumors were partially or totally cystic, and two were totally solid. All tumors but one had a suprasellar extension, which was responsible of the visual field defects. The mean size of the tumors' largest dimension was 29 mm (min 21, max 39). Preoperative open mouth CT scan revealed that all patients had a well-pneumatized sphenoid sinus (aka sellar type) and that the projection lines on the sella (see above) were divided into two presellar, three sellar, and two postsellar.

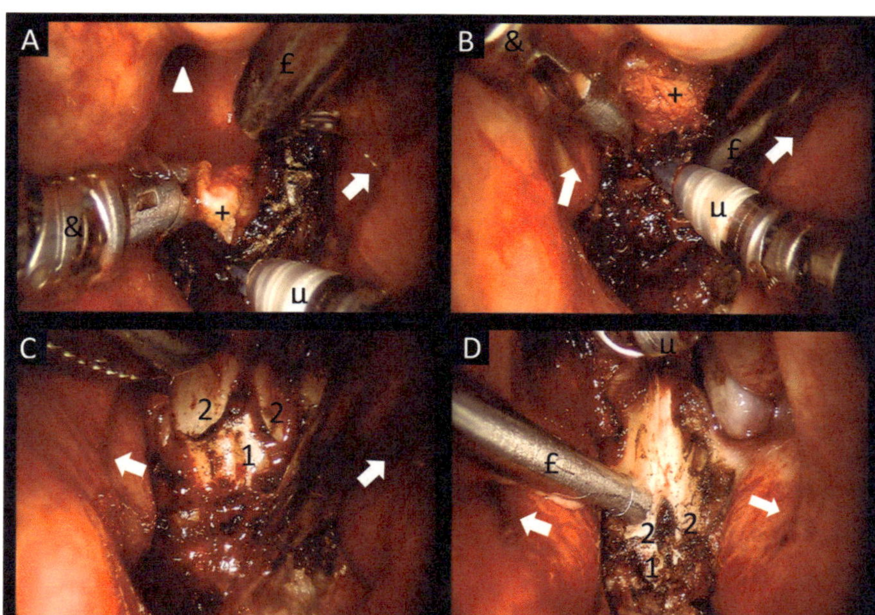

Figure 10. Intraoperative view at the console during mucosal time. (A and B) The mucosal flap (+) is progressively dissected and retracted upward using the Maryland dissector (&) and the monopolar cautery (µ) (patient n°1). (C) Visualization of the junction between the vomer, with its two alae (2), and the sphenoid bone (1) (patient n°1). (D) Suction (£) showing the key point to enter the sphenoid sinus (patient n°2). White triangle: right choanae; white arrows: Eustachian tubes [16].

Intraoperative data: the visualization of the cavum was good in all cases. However, we report one case in which the operative corridor was narrowed because of a thick mucosa. The mucosal flaps were dissected using the robot and reapplied at the end of surgery, except in one case as the flap was too retracted by the monopolar dissection. The key point at the junction between the vomer and the sphenoid was well identified in all cases (see **Figure 10**).

The sphenoid drilling allowed a penetration into the sphenoid sinus in all cases with a unique inferosuperior direction (see **Figure 11**).

The visualization of the sella was good, and the opening of the sella allowed reaching the tumor in all cases. Then, the removal quality depended on the tumor consistency. If the tumor was cystic (n = 5), the fluid drained off easily, and the curettage of solid component was quite easy. If the tumor was totally solid (n = 2), the removal was very hard because of two factors: (1) the surgery was very hemorrhagic, and we hypothesize that the position of the head was a possible reason; (2) the da Vinci system has no dedicated instruments such as curettes. This issue led to a partial removal, and patient n°5 had to be reoperated on via endonasal approach.

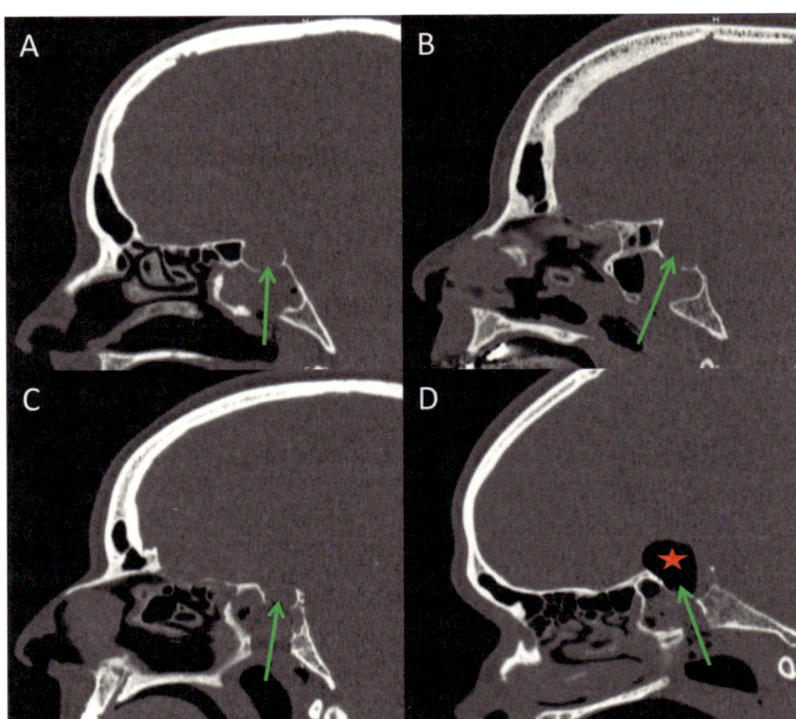

Figure 11. Postoperative brain CT scans at day 1 showing the inferosuperior approach of the sella with green arrows (A, B, C, and D for patients n°1, 2, 3, and 4, respectively). Red star indicates postoperative pneumocephalus in the pituitary fossa for patient n°4 [16].

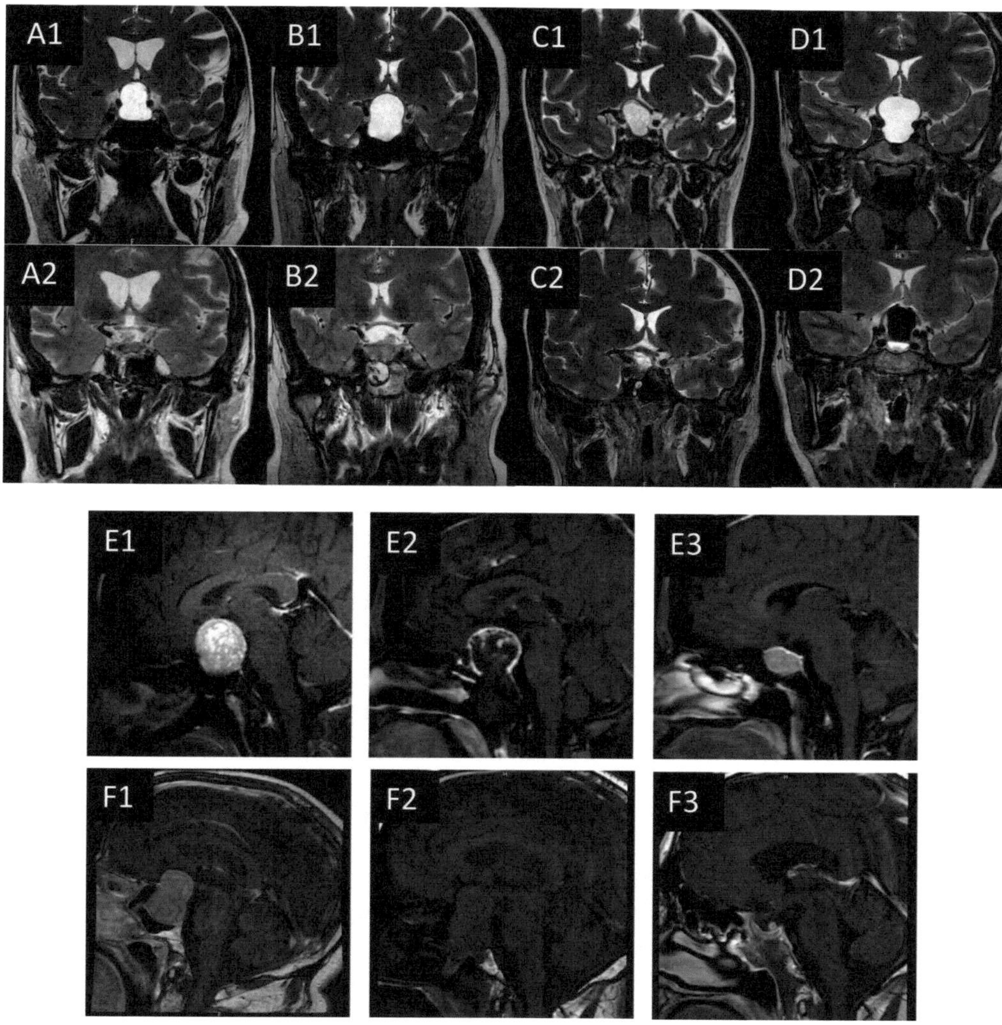

Figure 12. Upper figure shows coronal T2-weighted brain MR imagings, preoperatively (1) and postoperatively at day 1 (2). A, B, C, and D for patients n°1, 2, 3, and 4, respectively. For patient n°4, postoperative imaging (2D) shows intrasellar hyposignal corresponding to pneumocephalus [16]. Lower figure shows patient n°5 and 6, respectively, E and F. E1 preoperatively, E2 postoperatively at day 1 with hematoma within the sella, E3 postoperatively at 1 month with a resorption of the hematoma, and the chiasmatic decompression; F1 preoperatively, F2 postoperatively at day 1 with a partial reduction of the tumor, and F3 postoperatively after the second endonasal surgery.

At the end of the procedures, we observed three minor mucosal lip lesions (because of the drilling handpiece at the labial commissure) and two minor mucosal lesions next to the uvula (because of the loops to retract the soft palate).

Postoperative data: at 1 month after surgery, all patients have a better vision status. No rhinologic disturbance was noted. We reported the following TORS side effects: sore throat (n = 7) and hypernasal speech (n = 5). Fortunately, these symptoms were transient (approximately

3–5 days). One patient had an otitis media; we hypothesized that the reason could be a secondary constriction of the Eustachian tubes close to the dissected flap. We reported the following complications of sellar surgery: CSF leak (n = 1, resolved after lumbar puncture), diabetes insipidus (n = 2), and hypopituitarism (n = 1).

Regarding the postoperative MRI, we had good results about cystic lesions, but the removal quality was poor for the two solid tumors (see **Figure 12**).

Finally, we reported three pathological confirmations of gonadotroph adenomas. The other lesions were mainly cystic without diagnoses.

5. Conclusion

From this innovative TORS for sellar tumors, we can emphasize some promising results on cystic tumors, in a minimally invasive perspective because the side effects were minor and transient. The 3D visualization is very good, and the maneuverability of the robotic instruments is satisfying even in narrow spaces. Moreover, we think that this inferosuperior approach of the sella could bring interesting considerations for large suprasellar extension. However, we must comment on the lack of specific neurosurgical instruments in the da Vinci robot and the poor removal quality regarding solid pituitary adenomas, even if the tumors were reached in all cases.

Acknowledgements

We thank Prof. Lot for his general support regarding this project from the beginning to the last patients. We also thank Antoine Missistrano whose surgical assistance and general help were precious. We thank Wendy Gold for English corrections.

Conflict of interest

We declare no conflict.

Author details

Dorian Chauvet[1]* and Stephane Hans[2]

*Address all correspondence to: dchauvet@for.paris

1 Neurosurgery, Rothschild Foundation, Paris, France

2 Head and Neck Department, Hopital Européen George Pompidou, Paris, France

References

[1] Liu JK, Das K, Weiss MH, Laws ER Jr, Couldwell WT. The history and evolution of transsphenoidal surgery. Journal of Neurosurgery. 2001;**95**:1083-1096

[2] Yates DR, Vaessen C, Roupret M. From Leonardo to da Vinci: The history of robot-assisted surgery in urology. BJU International. 2011;**108**:1708-1713

[3] Advincula AP, Song A. The role of robotic surgery in gynecology. Current Opinion in Obstetrics & Gynecology. 2007;**19**:331-336

[4] Carrau RL, Prevedello DM, de Lara D, Durmus K, Ozer E. Combined transoral robotic surgery and endoscopic endonasal approach for the resection of extensive malignancies of the skull base. Head & Neck. 2013;**6**:351-358

[5] Hans S, Delas B, Gorphe P, Ménard M, Brasnu D. Transoral robotic surgery in head and neck cancer. European Annals of Otorhinolaryngology, Head and Neck Diseases. 2012;**129**(1):32-37

[6] Hans S, Hoffman C, Croidieu R, Vialatte de Pemille G, Crevier-Buchman L, Monfrais-Pfauwadel MC, et al. Evaluation of quality of life and swallowing in patients with cancer of the oropharynx treated with assisted transoral robotic surgery. Revue de Laryngologie Otologie Rhinologie. 2013;**134**:49-56

[7] Hans S, Jouffroy T, Veivers D, Hoffman C, Girod A, Badoual C, et al. Transoral robotic-assisted free flap reconstruction after radiation therapy in hypopharyngeal carcinoma: Report of two cases. European Archives of Oto-Rhino-Laryngology. 2013;**270**:2359-2364

[8] Lee JY, O'Malley BW, Newman JG, Weinstein GS, Lega B, Diaz J, et al. Transoral robotic surgery of craniocervical junction and atlantoaxial spine: A cadaveric study. Journal of Neurosurgery. Spine. 2010;**12**:13-18

[9] Lee JY, O'Malley BW Jr, Newman JG, Weinstein GS, Lega B, Diaz J, et al. Transoral robotic surgery of the skull base: A cadaver and feasibility study. ORL: Journal for Otorhinolaryngology and Its Related Specialties. 2010;**72**:181-187

[10] Yang MS, Yoon TH, Yoon DH, Kim KN, Pennant W, Ha Y. Robot-assisted transoral odontoidectomy: Experiment in new minimally invasive technology, a cadaveric study. Journal of Korean Neurosurgical Association. 2011;**49**:248-251

[11] Lee JY, Lega B, Bhowmick D, Newman JG, O'Malley BW Jr, Weinstein GS, et al. Da Vinci robot-assisted transoral odontoidectomy for basilar invagination. ORL: Journal for Otorhinolaryngology and Its Related Specialties. 2010;**72**:91-95

[12] Marcus HJ, Hughes-Hallett A, Cundy TP, Yang G-Z, Darzi A, Nandi D. Da Vinci robot-assisted keyhole neurosurgery: A cadaver study on feasibility and safety. Neurosurgical Review. 2015;**38**:367-371

[13] Crockard HA. The transoral approach to the base of the brain and upper cervical cord. Annals of the Royal College of Surgeons of England. 1985;**67**:321-325

[14] Chauvet D, Missistrano A, Hivelin M, Carpentier A, Cornu P, Hans S. Transoral robotic-assisted skull base surgery to approach the sella turcica: Cadaveric study. Neurosurgical Review. 2014;**37**:609-617

[15] Amelot A, Trunet S, Degos V, André O, Dionnet A, Cornu P, et al. Anatomical features of skull base and oral cavity: A pilot study to determine the accessibility of the sella by transoral robotic-assisted surgery. Neurosurgical Review. 2015;**38**:723-730

[16] Chauvet D, Hans S, Missistrano A, Rebours C, Bakourri WE, Lot G. Transoral robotic surgery for sellar tumors: First clinical study. Journal of Neurosurgery. 2017;**127**:941-948

[17] Hamberger CA, Hammer G, Marcusson G. Experiences in transantrosphenoidal hypophysectomy. Transactions of the Pacific Coast Oto-Ophthalmological Society Annual Meeting. 1961;**42**:273-286

Section 3

Pituitary Diseases

Chapter 4

Management of Celiac Patients with Growth Failure

Bozzola Mauro, Montalbano Chiara, Bozzola Elena,
Stamati Andreina Filomena, Larizza Daniela,
Ferrara Pietro and Villani Alberto

Additional information is available at the end of the chapter

http://dx.doi.org/10.5772/intechopen.77129

Abstract

Celiac disease (CD) may be considered as a systemic immune-mediated disorder that is triggered by dietary gluten in genetically susceptible subjects. CD children and adolescents show typical intestinal symptoms such as diarrhea, loss of weight and abdominal distension, or extraintestinal signs, the so-called nonclassical CD, such as short stature and delayed puberty. An endocrinological investigation including an evaluation of growth hormone (GH) secretion should be performed in CD subjects who show no catch-up growth after at least 1 year on a strict gluten-free diet (GFD) in the presence of a seronegativity of anti-transglutaminase and/or antiendomysial antibodies. When the diagnosis of GH deficiency is formulated, a substitutive therapy with GH must be promptly started to obtain a complete catch-up growth. The long-term effects of GH therapy in CD children who follow a strict GFD are comparable to those found in children with idiopathic GHD. A widely documented association has been observed between CD and type I diabetes mellitus and/or Hashimoto thyroiditis and/or Addison's disease. During follow-up, pediatricians should check antibody serology, thyroid and adrenal function and glucose-metabolic profile in order to verify the compliance with both diet and GH treatment. Adherence to a strict gluten-free diet promotes regular linear growth and may prevent CD complications as well as the onset of other autoimmune diseases.

Keywords: celiac disease, short stature, growth failure, growth hormone deficiency, growth hormone therapy

1. Introduction

Celiac disease (CD) may be considered as a systemic immune-mediated disorder that is triggered by the ingestion of dietary gluten in genetically susceptible subjects, resulting in various degrees of small intestinal damage.

Celiac disease affects approximately 1% of the population of Europe and North America, but it is estimated that the number of undiagnosed cases is currently far greater than that of diagnosed cases because of the presence of prevalent forms with nonspecific symptoms including short stature and delayed puberty [1, 2].

The clinical manifestation of celiac disease in children has changed over the last few years. The classic symptoms including diarrhea, growth failure and abdominal distension are becoming less common, and nonspecific signs and symptoms have become more frequent.

The various presentation of celiac disease ranges from typical gastrointestinal symptoms to extraintestinal signs, thus presenting the physician with a challenge in making an early diagnosis. It has been postulated that the diagnosis of celiac disease may be delayed by 3.5 years on average in patients who have extraintestinal symptoms [3].

Early diagnosis, especially in children, helps to reduce the impact of comorbidities and to increase final adult height [4, 5].

2. Celiac disease and short stature

Diagnosis of CD is based on serological testing for specific markers, such as circulating anti-transglutaminase and antiendomysial antibodies, and by histological analysis of duodenal biopsies.

A strict lifelong gluten-free diet (GFD) is the only effective treatment for celiac disease and usually results in a resolution of symptoms, disappearance of serum antibodies and repair of intestinal damage within 24 months. Full compliance to gluten-free diet reduces the risk of malignancy including T-cell lymphoma and non-Hodgkin's lymphoma [6].

When evaluating a child with short stature, the first step is to rule out celiac disease as short stature may be the only presenting symptom of the disease [7]. Between 8 and 10% of children with apparently idiopathic short stature have serologic evidence of celiac disease, i.e., positive IgA antibodies against tranglutaminase and anti-endomysium [8–11].

The probability of celiac disease in children with short stature of nonendocrinological cause is reported to be very high [12, 13].

For this reason, growth monitoring is very important for all children and, in particular, for those individuals with a higher risk of developing celiac disease. Population-based screening for celiac disease can be performed fairly accurately when several screening parameters for abnormal growth are used simultaneously, and combined with the use of longitudinal growth data [13].

The pathogenesis of growth failure is unclear. It is probably multifactorial and can be due to malabsorption, abnormalities in the endocrine hypothalamus-pituitary axis or growth hormone resistance [14].

Growth monitoring is a standard practice for a pediatrician. A child's height or length should be evaluated using specific devices. Children's length (for children less than 2 years old) is measured using a Harpenden infantometer. After the age of 2 years, height measurement requires the Harpenden stadiometer and the orthostatic position.

Growth percentile can be determined by correlating the child's height with their age on a growth chart. This practice is useful in comparing a patient's height to the expected parameters for children of the same age and sex. National and international growth charts report auxological parameters of a normal population from birth to adult age.

Growth charts are also useful in determining growth deceleration. Growth rate can be calculated using the difference between two height measurements detected in an at least period of 6–12 months. Growth rate below 10th percentile (or 25th for other authors) requires further diagnostic examinations.

No investigation of children's growth can be separated from the analysis of target height, which is determined by the measurement of the parents' height and the evaluation of pubertal development.

Weight evaluation and determination of BMI (body mass index) are essential in order to analyze children's growth. Weight and BMI should be reported on a specific growth chart [15].

In a celiac child with a stature below the 3rd percentile or below the percentile related to target height, a diagnostic work-up should be undertaken to investigate GH secretion. Diagnostic evaluation should be started immediately, without waiting for growth failure, if a CD subject shows the first pubertal signs, i.e., development of bud breast in females or increased testicular volume in males.

However, it is an accepted practice to rule out CD before evaluating GH secretion, since false GH responses to pharmacological stimuli have been observed, followed by their normalization after starting a GFD. It has been reported that 0.23% of children with short stature shows an association between CD and GH deficiency [10].

On the other hand, CD patients show catch-up growth generally after beginning the GFD and usually return to their normal growth within 1–2 years [16, 17].

Therefore, a careful follow-up is mandatory in order to verify the normal growth progression, as well as annual evaluation of serology negativity. If the CD subject does not show catch-up growth, and tests negative for "celiac" antibodies, an evaluation of GH secretion is mandatory [17].

In the event of GH deficiency confirmed by a serum peak response of less than 8 ng/ml to at least two pharmacological stimuli, and in the presence of negative serologic tests for anti-transglutaminase antibodies, substitutive GH therapy should be started.

GH basal levels are normally very low and they are not useful in confirming GH deficiency.

GH secretion may be not so easy to measure because it is regulated by different peptides and neurotransmitters, such as GHRH and somatostatin, and it is pulsatile throughout the day. Given the poor reproducibility and accuracy of these tests, clinicians should bear in mind that GHD diagnosis is based on clinical and auxological findings that suggest a hypothesis of GHD [18].

The results of stimulation tests serve merely to confirm the clinical diagnosis.

Spontaneous and stimulated GH secretion is variable. Levels vary significantly according to gender, age, weight and pubertal status [19].

Moreover, spontaneous GH secretion progressively decreases with age, and this trend is more pronounced in males. During the pubertal period, there is a marked increase in GH secretion, which is directly influenced by sex steroids. Where there is an increase in body mass index, a decreasing trend of GH peak values after stimulation tests has been observed.

However, in clinical practice, a specific range based on age, sex, weight and pubertal stage does not exist.

Serum GH cut-off values for pharmacological stimulation tests depend on the type of stimulus and the method used for determining serum GH.

For this reason, there are specific recommendations within guidelines aimed at standardizing GH assays [20].

In clinical practice, stimulation tests include different pharmacological stimuli. Given the poor reproducibility of these tests, it has been established that two provocative tests are required for a diagnosis of GH deficiency.

Provocative tests should be performed in pediatric endocrinology centers with experienced teams; particular attention is required when administering insulin and glucagon, due to the risk of symptomatic hypoglycemia.

The insulin tolerance test (ITT) is considered the gold standard in evaluating GH secretion. Insulin-induced hypoglycemia acts as a stimulus for GH secretion. Insulin is administered intravenously (0.1 unit/kg in children over 4 years of age and 0.05 unit/kg in younger children). Then blood samples are collected to measure GH, glucose and cortisol levels, at 0, 30, 60, 90, 120 minutes after insulin injection. This test requires careful observation by experienced staff because of the risk of hypoglycemia. If the blood glucose level decreases by 40–50% of basal value or reaches less than 40 mg/dl, the test is considered effective. Usually, GH peak occurs 15–30 minutes after glucose nadir.

Glucagon induces GH secretion by stimulating endogenous insulin secretion following an increase in blood glucose level. It is administered intramuscularly (0.03 mg/kg, maximum 1 mg). Measurements of GH, cortisol and glucose are carried out after 30, 60, 120, 150, and 180 minutes after glucagon administration. GH peak is usually observed after 2–3 hours (concurrently with hypoglycemia).

Arginine inhibits somatostatin release. The arginine provocative test consists of IV infusion of arginine hydrochloride (0.5 g/kg, maximum 40 g) over a 30-minute period. Blood samples should be collected at baseline and after 30, 60, 90, and 120 minutes after infusion. GH peak is expected to occur 60 minutes after arginine administration.

GHRH can directly assess pituitary gland capacity to secrete GH. The GHRH test (alone or in combination with arginine administration) is useful in diagnosing hypothalamic defects. A dosage of 1 mcg/kg of GHRH is administered intravenously. Serum samples are collected at baseline and 15, 30, 45, 60, 90, and 120 minutes after GHRH administration (frequently with concurrent infusion of arginine hydrochloride). GHRH plus arginine stimulates GH secretion to a greater extent than GHRH alone. The GHRH plus arginine test is useful for identifying false-positive GH deficiency in children with blunted GH secretion after the classic pharmacological provocative tests [21] (**Table 1**).

IGFs (insulin-like growth factors) are GH-dependent peptides that mediate many of the anabolic and mitogenic actions of GH. IGF-1 and IGF-binding protein-3 (IGFBP-3) levels depend on GH secretion. Given the stability of its serum levels during the day, the measurement of serum IGF-1 should be a useful tool in evaluating GH secretion, bypassing provocation tests and their poor reproducibility. IGF-1 levels are influenced by age and pubertal development and, although age and puberty-corrected IGF-1 reference values have been generated, an overlap between IGF-1 values for normal and GHD children still exists, particularly in children younger than 5 years of age. Serum IGF-1 levels can vary between laboratories due to the different assay methods used. Most investigators have used cutoffs of either the 5th percentile or less than −2 SD to define subnormal levels of IGF-1 [22].

Guidelines consider a value of IGF-1 below 0 SD as an indication to undergo provocative tests. In fact, individuals with idiopathic GHD and a serum IGF-1 level of greater than 0 SD for age are highly likely to have normal provocative tests [20].

IGF-1 levels are also influenced by nutritional conditions: reduced IGF-1 levels may occur in children with malnutrition. Low IGF-1 serum values are described in case of hypothyroidism, hepatic disease and diabetes.

IGFBP-3 values are also used in the diagnostic approach to GHD, but no correlation has been found between GH levels and serum levels of IGFBP-3 in assessing GHD.

Although low serum levels of IGF-1 and IGFBP-3 would suggest a diagnosis of GH deficiency (given the mechanism of action of GH), normal levels do not rule out the possibility of GHD. Therefore, we should perform a provocative test as recommended by the guidelines of the Pediatric Endocrine Society [20].

Low levels of insulin-like growth factor 1 and insulin-like growth factor binding protein (IGFBP) are reported in patients with CD [23].

Stimulus	Dosage
Insulin (ITT) IV	0.05–0.1 U/kg (max 4 U)
Glucagon IM	0.03 mg/kg (max 1 mg)
Arginine hydrochloride IV	0.5 g/kg (max 40 g)
GHRH IV	1 mcg/kg

ITT: insulin tolerance test; IV: intravenously; IM: intramuscular; GHRH: growth hormone-releasing hormone.

Table 1. Growth hormone provocative tests.

Treatment with rhGH should be started as soon as possible after the diagnosis, with a view to obtaining normalization of height during childhood and a better adult height.

Before starting GH treatment, it is necessary to check glucose tolerance (by performing an oral glucose tolerance test, named OGTT) because growth hormone may contribute to insulin resistance.

Especially in cases of total deficiency (GH peak <4 ng/ml), possible deficiencies of other pituitary hormones including TSH, ACTH, FSH, LH should be investigated.

In the rare cases of GHD associated with a deficiency of one or more pituitary hormones, adequate hormonal secretion should be restored by substitutive therapy before starting GH therapy. The doses of the missing hormones such as levothyroxine, hydrocortisone, estradiol, testosterone and desmopressin, are the same as those used in idiopathic GHD patients.

A deficiency in pituitary gonadotropins, LH and FSH, can be assessed only during puberty when an increase in pubertal gonadotropin occurs.

Brain magnetic resonance may be required to rule out morphological hypothalamus-pituitary region abnormalities.

CD patients with GHD should be treated with the same GH dosage utilized in patients with idiopathic GHD. Substitutive therapy should be started at the weekly dosage of 0.25 mg/kg divided in six daily subcutaneous injections administered in the evening before sleeping to mimic the physiological night-time elevation of spontaneous GH [24].

International protocols suggest increasing the dosage and/or administering therapy every day during puberty, without a weekly rest, to maximize growth during this period [20].

Subcutaneous administration is the best delivery procedure due to ease of execution and good patient compliance. It is necessary to vary the injection site to avoid lipodystrophy, which may prevent GH absorption. If properly motivated and instructed, the child may administer the GH therapy himself.

GH treatment should be monitored every 6 months by evaluating the biomarkers of thyroid function such as FT4 and TSH, adrenal function such as cortisol basal values, and the glucose-metabolic profile including blood glucose, glycated hemoglobin and insulin basal levels.

Recently, monitoring IGF-I every 6 months has been suggested since it may evaluate adherence to treatment and help clinicians modify GH dosage in order to optimize growth response.

If serum IGF-1 levels exceed the normal value for age or pubertal stage, reducing the GH dose is recommended [20].

If catch-up growth does not occur, it is necessary to suspend treatment and reconsider diagnosis. Anti-GH antibodies should be evaluated, although their occurrence is very rare in clinical practice.

Both height and growth velocity significantly improves during GH therapy, confirming that catch-up growth following GFD is due to low GH secretion. The growth velocity increases especially during the first year of GH therapy, and subsequently remains constant, although always above pre-treatment values [17].

The long-term effects of GH therapy in CD children who follow a strict GFD are comparable to those found in children with idiopathic GHD. During follow-up, pediatricians should check antibody serology, thyroid and adrenal function and the glucose-metabolic profile in order to verify the compliance with both diet and GH treatment.

The height CD subjects attain in adulthood does not differ from that of idiopathic GHD patients. Adherence to a strict gluten-free diet plays an important role in the management of celiac disease leading to a good response to GH treatment [24].

Patients with GH deficiency in childhood are usually re-tested in late adolescence or young adulthood because GHD may persist into adult life. A provocative test is repeated after at least 1 month of GH-therapy washout. It is possible to use a GHRH plus arginine test (a value >19 ng/ml is considered normal) or insulin tolerance test (ITT), considering a value of up to 6 ng/ml as normal secretion. No other tests have been validated for re-evaluation of the somatotropic axis [25].

When a diagnosis of adult GHD is established, continuation of GH therapy is recommended. The growth hormone is involved in numerous ongoing metabolic processes in adult life.

In the presence of a normal GH response to at least one pharmacological stimulus, the auxological follow-up should continue until adult age. Careful clinical surveillance is mandatory: if patient presents growth failure is necessary to repeat auxological evaluation.

Furthermore, CD must be ruled out also in subjects with delayed appearance of pubertal signs, i.e., in girls over 13 years old with an absence of mammary glands and in boys over 14 years old with a testicular volume of less than 4 ml.

Delayed puberty may be one of the extraintestinal manifestations of celiac disease. Delayed menarche has been documented in girls with CD but not in those on a gluten-free diet.

In males, androgen resistance has been implicated in the development of celiac disease. The exact correlation between CD and delayed puberty is not known. Autoimmunity directed against hormonal axis has been proposed as a causative mechanism. Furthermore, it has been suggested that malabsorption of micronutrients may influence hormone synthesis [26, 27].

Other reasons for nonresponse may be due to less-than-strict adherence to GFD or other underlying comorbidities including diabetes mellitus type I and Hashimoto thyroiditis. Thus, re-evaluation of the compliance to GFD or research for additional underlying comorbidities in CD patients failing to respond to GFD is mandatory.

3. Conclusions

In children presenting with short stature, the first step should be to rule out subclinical hypothyroidism and celiac disease before referring them for other endocrine tests.

On the other hand, careful assessment of growth rate and pubertal development is mandatory in children diagnosed as celiac on the basis of serological testing for specific markers and histological analysis of duodenal biopsies. Normal growth velocity does not require further endocrine tests. However, in cases of growth velocity deceleration under the 10th–25th percentile, thyroid function must be evaluated to exclude Hashimoto thyroiditis. Subsequently, an evaluation of GH secretion in CD patients should be requested mainly if no catch-up growth is observed within 1 year on a strict GFD and in those whose tests are negative for anti-transglutaminase and anti-endomysium antibodies.

Moreover, in CD subjects with GHD, substitutive GH therapy should be promptly started and administered at standard doses daily in order to achieve complete catch-up growth.

The long-time effects of GH therapy in children who follow a strict diet are similar to those observed in children with idiopathic GHD. Finally, during follow-up, the clinician must carefully verify adherence to GFD and check seronegativity, auxological parameters, thyroid and adrenal function, and glucose-metabolic profile. Before deciding whether to interrupt or continue GH therapy in a patient who has reached definitive stature, hormonal secretion retesting is needed in order to identify patients at risk of developing adult deficiency.

Acknowledgements

The authors are grateful to Sheila McVeigh for the English revision of the manuscript. The authors would like to acknowledge the Adolfo Ferrata Medicine Library Staff of the University of Pavia (Italy) for their invaluable assistance and irreplaceable help.

Conflict of interest

The authors declare no conflict of interest.

Author details

Bozzola Mauro[1,2]*, Montalbano Chiara[1], Bozzola Elena[3], Stamati Andreina Filomena[4], Larizza Daniela[1], Ferrara Pietro[5] and Villani Alberto[3]

*Address all correspondence to: mauro.bozzola@unipv.it

1 Department of Internal Medicine and Therapeutics, Unit of Pediatrics and Adolescentology, University of Pavia, Pavia, Italy

2 Onlus "Il Bambino e il suo pediatra", Galliate, Novara, Italy

3 Department of Pediatrics, Pediatric and Infectious Diseases Unit, Bambino Gesù Children Hospital IRCCS, Rome, Italy

4 Unit of Pediatrics and Neonatology, Ferrari Hospital, Castrovillari, Cosenza, Italy

5 Catholic University, Institute of Pediatrics, Rome, Italy

References

[1] Fasano A, Berti I, Gerarduzzi T, Not T, Colletti RB, Drago S, Elitsur Y, Green PH, Guandalini S, Hill ID, Pietzak M, Ventura A, Thorpe M, Kryszak D, Fornaroli F, Wasserman SS, Murray JA, Horvath K. Prevalence of celiac disease in at-risk and not-at-risk groups in the United States: A large multicenter study. Archives of Internal Medicine. 2003;**163**:286-292

[2] Lionetti E, Catassi C. New clues in celiac disease epidemiology, pathogenesis, clinical manifestations, and treatment. International Reviews of Immunology. 2011;**30**:219-231

[3] Paez MA, Gramelspacher AM, Sinacore J, Winterfield L, Venu M. Delay in diagnosis of celiac disease in patients without gastrointestinal complaints. The American Journal of Medicine. 2017;**130**:1318-1323

[4] Craig D, Fayter D, Stirk L, Crott R. Growth monitoring for short stature: Update of a systematic review and economic model. Health Technology Assessment. 2011 Feb;**15**(11: iii-iv):1-64

[5] Grote FK, van Dommelen P, Oostdijk W, et al. Developing evidence-based guidelines for referral for short stature. Archives of Disease in Childhood. 2008;**93**:212-217

[6] Green PH, Fleischauer AT, Bhagat G, Goyal R, Jabri B, Neugut AI. Risk of malignancy in patients with celiac disease. The American Journal of Medicine. 2003;**115**:191-195

[7] Meazza C, Pagani S, Laarej K, Cantoni F, Civallero P, Boncimino A, Bozzola M. Short stature in children with coeliac disease. Pediatric Endocrinology Reviews. 2009;**6**:457-463

[8] Rosenbach Y, Dinari G, Zahavi I, Nitzan M. Short stature as the major manifestation of coeliac disease in older children. Clinical Pediatrics (Phila). 1986;**25**:13-16

[9] Stenhammar L, Fallstrom SP, Jansson G, Jansson U, Lindberg T. Coeliac disease in children with short stature without gastrointestinal symptoms. European Journal of Pediatrics. 1986;**145**:185-186

[10] Bonamico M, Scirè G, Mariani P, Pasquino AM, Triglione P, Scaccia S, Ballati G, Boscherini B. Short stature as the primary manifestation of monosymptomatic celiac disease. Journal of Pediatric Gastroenterology and Nutrition. 1992;**14**:12-16

[11] Giovenale D, Meazza C, Cardinale GM, Sposito M, Mastrangelo C, Messini B, Citro G, Delvecchio M, di Maio S, Bozzola M. The prevalence of growth hormone deficiency and celiac disease in short children. Clinical Medicine & Research. 2006;**4**:180-183

[12] JC v R, Grote FK, Oostdijk W, Wit JM. Short stature and the probability of coeliac disease, in the absence of gastrointestinal symptoms. Archives of Disease in Childhood. 2004 Sep;**89**(9):882-883

[13] Saari A, Harju S, Mäkitie O, Saha M, Dunkel L, Sankilampi U. Systematic growth monitoring for the early detection of celiac disease in children. JAMA Pediatrics. 2015;**169**(3): e1525

[14] Troncone R, Kosova R. Short stature and catch-up growth in celiac disease. Journal of Pediatric Gastroenterology and Nutrition. 2010;**51**(suppl 3):S137-S138

[15] Christesen HT, Pedersen BT, Pournara E, Petit IO, Júlíusson PB. Short stature: Comparison of WHO and national growth standards/references for height. PLoS One. 2016;**11**(6): e0157277

[16] Knudtzon J, Fluge G, Aksnes L. Routine measurements of gluten antibodies in children of short stature. Journal of Pediatric Gastroenterology and Nutrition. 1991;**12**:190-194

[17] Bozzola M, Giovenale D, Bozzola E, Meazza C, Martinetti M, Tinelli C, Corazza GR. Growth hormone deficiency and coeliac disease: An unusual association? Clinical Endocrinology. 2005;**62**:372-375

[18] Obara-Moszynska M, Kedzia A, Korman E, Niedziela M. Usefulness of growth hormone (GH) stimulation tests and IGF-1 concentration measurement in GH deficiency diagnosis. Journal of Pediatric Endocrinology & Metabolism. 2008;**21**:569-579

[19] Richmond EJ, Rogol AD. Growth hormone deficiency in children. Pituitary. 2008;**11**(2): 115-120

[20] Grimberg A, DiVall SA, Polychronakos C, Allen DB, Cohen LE, Quintos JB, Rossi WC, Feudtner C, Murad MH. Drug and therapeutics committee and ethics committee of the pediatric endocrine society. Guidelines for growth hormone and insulin-like growth Factor-1 treatment in children and adolescents: Growth hormone deficiency, idiopathic short stature, and primary insulin-like growth factor-I deficiency. Hormone Research in Pædiatrics. 2016;**86**:361-397

[21] Mazzola A, Meazza C, Travaglino P, Pagani S, Frattini D, Bozzola E, Corneli G, Aimaretti G, Bozzola M. Unreliability of classic provocative tests for the diagnosis of growth hormone deficiency. Journal of Endocrinological Investigation. 2008 Feb;**31**(2):159-162

[22] Badaru A, Wilson DM. Alternatives to growth hormone stimulation testing in children. Trends in Endocrinology and Metabolism. 2004 Aug;**15**(6):252-258

[23] Locuratolo N, Pugliese G, Pricci F, Romeo G, Mariani P, Diaz-Horta O, Calvani L, Montuori M, Cipolletta E, Di Mario U, Bonamico M. The circulating insulin-like growth factor system in children with coeliac disease: An additional marker for disease activity. Diabetes/metabolism Research and Reviews. 1999 Jul-Aug;**15**(4):254-260

[24] Meazza C, Pagani S, Messini B, Cardinale GM, Mastrangelo C, Citro G, Delvecchio M, Tinelli C, Corazza GR, Bozzola M. Celiac children treated for growth hormone deficiency reach normal final height. Clinical Endocrinology. 2011;**74**:791-792

[25] Gasco V, Corneli G, Beccuti G, et al. Retesting the childhood-onset GH-deficient patient. European Journal of Endocrinology. 2008;**159**:S45-S52

[26] Bona G, Marinello D, Oderda G. Mechanisms of abnormal puberty in coeliac disease. Hormone Research. 2002;**57**(Suppl 2):63-65

[27] Leffler DA, Green PH, Fasano A. Extraintestinal manifestations of coeliac disease. Reviews Gastroenterology and Hepatology. 2015 Oct;**12**(10):561-571

Chapter 5

Pituitary Apoplexy

Manel Jemel, Wafa Alaya, Fedia Boubaker,
Olfa Berrich and Baha Zantour

Additional information is available at the end of the chapter

http://dx.doi.org/10.5772/intechopen.77270

Abstract

Pituitary apoplexy is a rare clinical emergency due to acute ischemic infarction or hemorrhage of the pituitary gland. As this disorder most often involves a pituitary adenoma, especially nonfunctioning tumors, the syndrome should be referred to as pituitary tumor apoplexy. The precise physiopathology is not completely clear. Although in most cases it occurs spontaneously, pituitary apoplexy can be precipitated by many risk factors. The main symptom is headache of sudden onset associated with visual disturbances, signs of meningeal irritation, and/or endocrine dysfunction. Corticotropic deficiency is a potentially life-threatening disorder. Magnetic resonance imaging is the most sensitive to confirm the diagnosis by revealing a pituitary tumor with hemorrhagic and/or necrotic components. Earlier studies used to consider urgent decompression of the lesion surgically, but nowadays, more recent studies favor conservative management in selected patients (those without important visual acuity or field defects and with normal consciousness). This wait-and-see approach gives evidence of excellent outcomes in terms of oculomotor palsy, pituitary function, and subsequent tumor growth. Surgical decompression may be necessary in some cases. Once the acute phase is over, the patient should be reevaluated for hormonal deficiencies. Moreover, spontaneous remission of syndromes, such as acromegaly, may be caused by pituitary adenoma apoplexy.

Keywords: apoplexy, hypopituitarism, pituitary adenoma, pituitary MRI

1. Introduction

The term "pituitary apoplexy" (PA) originating from Greek means "sudden attack" with hemorrhage and/or infarction in the pituitary tumor or, less commonly, the surrounding normal gland tissue.

The first index case was, described by Bailey, in 1898 [1], but the term pituitary apoplexy was coined by Broughamin in 1950 [2].

Pituitary tumor apoplexy is an uncommon acute clinical syndrome and one of the rare problems that is diagnostically and therapeutically challenging.

PA is frequently the onset of unknown preexisting pituitary adenoma. The clinical spectrum of presentation does vary but often reserved only for classical presentation in contrast to "Silent, subclinical or asymptomatic pituitary tumor apoplexy" even though the latter is the more frequent entity [3].

It is a potentially life-threatening complication requiring a rapid diagnosis and appropriate treatment.

The diagnosis of pituitary tumor apoplexy is based on imaging evaluations, mainly using magnetic resonance imaging.

The best approach in the acute phase is still controversial, and nowadays, PA is no longer considered as a neurosurgical emergency [4, 5].

The outcome of acute apoplexy is variable and remains difficult to predict; a regular input and follow-up from a multidisciplinary team including neurosurgeons, endocrinologists, neuro-ophthalmologists, neuroradiologists, and neurologists are mandatory.

2. Epidemiological data

Pituitary tumor apoplexy appears to be rare. The true incidence and prevalence of PA are difficult to establish either because the majority of the studies are retrospectives or because the diagnosis of PA is usually misdiagnosed and simply identified at surgery or during radiological investigation or pathological examination. According to the main retrospective series, an estimated prevalence of 6.2 cases per 100,000 inhabitants and [6] an incidence of 0.17 episodes per 100,000 person-years were reported [7].

In published series of surgically resected pituitary adenomas, PA can occur in 0.6–10% with a mean of 2% of all adenomas and has reached 21% in an unusual report [8]. Nonfunctioning pituitary adenomas (NFPA) appear to be at higher risk of apoplexy with an incidence of 0.2–0.6 events per 100 person-years [9]. In published series of nonfunctioning pituitary adenomas, the frequency of apoplexy can vary from 3.7 to 21% [10]. Nonsecreting pituitary adenomas represent an average of 45–70% of adenomas with apoplexy [3].

Apoplexy represents the first clinical manifestation of previously unknown pituitary adenoma in 60–80% of cases [5, 11, 12].

Pituitary tumor apoplexy can occur at all ages, but most cases are seen during the fifth or sixth decade of life. In adolescents, this event has been described by Jankoswski and cols as a very rare entity [13].

There is a discrete preponderance in males ranging from 1.1 to 2.3/1 [5, 12].

Macroadenomas, especially nonfunctioning, and prolactinomas are most susceptible to apoplexy; nevertheless, apoplexy in other tumor types such as GH-secreting or clinically silent ACTH adenomas has been reported [5].

Microadenomas may also be prone to apoplexy [14]. PA occurs in 0.6–10% of treated pituitary adenomas. In three series of macroprolactinomas, the ratio of apoplexy/therapy varied between 1.2 and 6.67% [14].

In a review, apoplexy was found to occur in 1–6% of macroprolactinomas. This average was comparable between treated and untreated adenomas [5].

Semple et al. have found that one-third of their 62 patients had only infarction [15]. Hemorrhage is more associated with macroprolactinoma and female gender [16].

3. Pathophysiology

The pathophysiological mechanisms of pituitary tumor apoplexy remain incompletely understood. There are various theories upon the pathophysiology of pituitary apoplexy in the current literature. It is uncertain whether the pathological process is a primary hemorrhage or whether the event is really a hemorrhagic infarction. Many pathogenic mechanisms have been proposed. Given that the risk of hemorrhage in a pituitary adenoma appears to be five times higher than in other intracranial neoplasms, intrinsic factors can be involved in the apoplectic event [12]. The rich and the complex vascular system makes the pituitary adenomas more vulnerable to bleed than any other brain tumor.

Understanding the vascularity of the pituitary gland and pituitary adenomas is crucial for etiopathogenesis of apoplexy.

As shown by the angiographic studies, the adenomas are mostly supplied by inferior pituitary artery, and its arterial flux is reduced compared with the normal pituitary [17].

The number and size of vessels are generally lesser than the normal pituitary vessels and are divided into irregular islets. Under electronic microscopy, they have incomplete maturation, poor fenestration, and ruptured and fragmented basal membranes with perivascular spaces filled with plasmatic proteins or red cells that may predispose to hemorrhage [18].

The fragility of the constitutional tumoral vascularization, can be explained by an increased expression of vascular endothelial growth factor "VEGF mRNA" in pituitary tumors; especially in nonfunctioning pituitary adenomas [14].

This expression of vascular endothelial growth factor could be explained by a tumoral overexpression of the pituitary tumor transforming and was found to correlate positively with the risk of pituitary hemorrhage. Other vascular markers were reported such as fetal liver kinase 1, nestin, etc. [5].

All the conditions associated with an acute increase in blood flow or coagulation disturbs may predispose these lesions to hemorrhage or hemorrhagic infarction [14].

This intratumoural vasculopathy, limited blood supply of the pituitary adenomas, and limited expression of angiogenic factors contrast with a high-energy requirement. As consequence, any extrinsic factor that alters the balance between tumor perfusion and tumor metabolism may cause an acute ischemia or infarction [17].

Moreover, an increased intratumoural and intrasellar pressure could concur to the reduction of tumor perfusion, further contributing to ischemia's pathomechanisms. Tumor growth could thus contribute to ischemia which explains the size of the adenoma being a major factor. Macroadenomas are described to be at a much higher risk of apoplexy than microadenomas [10, 19, 20].

Germline AIP gene mutations may be associated with a rapid growth of the pituitary adenomas predisposing them to apoplexy [21].

4. Predisposing factors

PA can occur without any risk factors; however, numerous conditions have been linked to PA. Precipitating factors are identified in 10–40% of cases [3] (**Table 1**).

4.1. Precipitating factors

The multiple factors reported as precipitating PA can be classified into three categories.

4.1.1. Acute variations of the blood flow in the pituitary gland

Procedures such as angiography, pneumoencephalography, myelography, lumbar puncture, and spinal anesthesia have been associated with PA. Blood pressure (BP) fluctuations or vasospasm may explain PA [22, 23]. Pituitary irradiation may induce vascular changes leading to chronic hypoperfusion of the pituitary gland and has been associated with both pituitary infarction and pituitary hemorrhage [24, 25]. Closed-head trauma which often minor may be a cause of PA, explained by acute changes in the intracranial pressure and in blood pressure [26].

Precipitating factors
Major surgery: coronary artery bypass surgery
Coronary artery bypass grafting/stenting
Coagulopathies, anticoagulation, thrombolytic and antiplateled Therapy
Clotting disorder
Dynamic endocrine stimulation testing with TRH, GNRH,
Estrogen therapy
Medications: Dopamine agonist therapy, GnRH agonist
Systemic hypertension/hypotension
Head trauma
Radiotherapy
Pregnancy

Table 1. Precipitating factors of pituitary apoplexy.

PA has been described in postoperative states. Orthopedic and cardiac surgeries mainly cardiopulmonary bypass were the most incriminated [27–29]. Intra- or postoperative hypotension, anticoagulation, and microemboli leading to infarction were the proposed mechanisms. If a pituitary adenoma is known before the cardiac procedure, some authors recommend the use of off-pump technique maintaining an adequate systemic perfusion, as opposed to standard cardiopulmonary bypass [30].

Systemic hypertension leading to an increase in blood flow and diabetes mellitus has been associated with PA [31, 32]. However, this association was not confirmed by other studies [10, 33].

Severe vomiting/diarrhea with concomitant increased Valsalva pressure may also decrease blood supply to the pituitary adenoma and precipitate apoplexy, since tumoral cells are particularly sensitive to glucose deprivation [5].

4.1.2. Imbalance between the stimulation of the pituitary and the ability of increased blood flow at the level of the pituitary adenoma

Apoplexy can also occur after dynamic testing of the pituitary (insulin, TRH, GnRH, or GHRH tests and much more rarely CRH) particularly when different agents are combined. Numerous publications have documented the occurrence of apoplexy within minutes to hours after testing [10, 34, 35].

In this setting, TRH dynamic test may cause apoplexy by vasospasm induced by increased norepinephrine levels or by elevating systemic pressure.

Other tests of pituitary stimulation (especially use of GnRH) can increase the imbalance between the intratumoral metabolic demand and the poor tumor perfusion.

Reports of PA occurring after stimulation test are much rarer in the recent past. Currently, pituitary dynamic testing is not commonly used in the routine assessment of hypothalamic pituitary function.

Increased estrogen states, such as exogenous estrogen administration, pregnancy, and postpartum period, have been reported to cause PA [33, 36–38]. Treatment with GnRH agonists for prostate cancer has also been associated with PA [39–41].

The role of dopamine agonist (DAs) treatment as precipitating factor is more controversial, although many case reports suggested this hypothesis [42, 43]. In prospective studies analyzing the effects of DAs on macroprolactinomas, PA were very rarely or never observed [6, 44–46]. In a retrospective study [9], DA treatment of pituitary adenomas was not associated with PA. These results are not surprising, given that these agents decrease growth and activity of prolactinoma or other adenoma cells.

PA can occur in the setting of an acute systemic illness such as myocardial infarction or severe infection. Excessive stimulation of the pituitary gland by production of larger amount of steroids is a possible explanation [33].

4.1.3. Anticoagulated states

PA has been observed after administration of anticoagulant drugs (vitamin K antagonist or platelet inhibitors) or thrombolytic agents, sometimes very soon after the initiation of treatment or after a prolonged period of treatment [6, 9, 47]. New classes of anticoagulant (dabigatran) [48, 49] may also be involved.

Thrombocytopenia has also been reported usually associated with hemorrhagic PA [50, 51].

4.2. Influence of pituitary adenoma type

The prevalence of apoplexy according to different subtypes of pituitary tumors shows a trend for nonfunctioning adenomas [3–5, 9, 22, 33, 52–55] to develop apoplexy. It is believed that nonfunctioning tumors may be diagnosed at a later stage, so they grow to a larger size before diagnosis; in contrast, the functioning adenomas are generally revealed earlier by signs of hormonal secretion before bleeding/infarction occurs [5].

Other tumor types predisposing to apoplexy are prolactinomas and GH-secreting adenomas [27, 56–59]. In the vast majority of cases, apoplexy complicates large macroadenomas [10]. Clinically silent ACTH adenomas may be particularly prone to necrosis, hemorrhage, and cyst transformation [5, 60]. These complications occur in 30–64% of cases, 2–14% in patients with all types of pituitary adenoma [16, 61–63].

5. Clinical presentation

Frequently, the PA episode is the first manifestation of undiagnosed pituitary adenoma [22, 57, 64].

It is important to consider that the pituitary apoplexy has a wide spectrum of clinical features, resulting from undergoing sudden mass enlargement. It ranges from silent asymptomatic necrotic and/or hemorrhagic adenoma to "classic" acute presentation and even death.

This is largely depending on the extent of hemorrhage, necrosis, and edema. Semple et al. suggested that the cases of pituitary tumor infarction alone had less severe clinical features and better outcome than those with hemorrhagic infarction or frank hemorrhage [15].

The clinical manifestations are summarized in **Table 2**.

5.1. Neurologic symptoms

Headache is the earliest and most common presenting symptom with an incidence of more than 90% [4, 65, 66].

The cephalalgia onset is often sudden and severe, namely, "thunderclap headache," in patients presenting with pituitary apoplexy and creates an even greater degree of difficulty in the differential diagnoses. It is usually resistant to analgesics, mainly retro-orbital and sometimes http://dx.doi.org/10.5772/intechopen.77270

Clinical presentation
Sudden onset headache
Vomiting, nausea
Photophobia
Meningism
Visual field and acuity defects
Diplopia/opthalmoplegia
Pyrexia
Cranial nerve palsy
Third nerve (more frequent)
Fourth nerve (trochlear)
Fifth nerve (1st and 2nd branches of trigeminal)
Sixth nerve (abducens)
Altered mental status
Seizure
Reduced conscious level
Facial pain/impaired facial sensation
Collapse
Hemiparesis
Sudden Death

Table 2. Common clinical features of pituitary apoplexy.

bifrontal, suboccipital, or diffuse [67]. This feature can be explained by meningeal irritation due to extravasation of blood and necrotic material into subarachnoid space, enlargement of sella turcica walls, dura mater compression, or involvement of the superior division of the trigeminal nerve inside the cavernous sinus [18, 68].

Headache is commonly accompanied by signs of meningeal irritation, such as nausea and vomiting (57%), photophobia (40%), meningismus (25%), and fever (16%) [5]. The fifth cranial nerve (first branch) can be involved in PA, resulting in facial numbness [3].

Altered level of consciousness may occur in varying degrees ranging from lethargy to stupor or even coma as consequence of blood or necrotic tissue leaking into the subarachnoid space [69]. A concurrent cerebrovascular episode with a stroke has been previously described [70]. The involvement of the thalamus in a case of pituitary apoplexy with thalamic and midbrain infarction has been described [71]. In such cases, one of the following mechanisms was proposed: (1) compression of intracavernous portion of internal carotid artery due to expanding pituitary adenoma or a hemorrhage within it and (2) vasospasm caused by factors released from hemorrhagic or necrotic material [70].

Rare cases of sudden death following pituitary tumor apoplexy of fatal outcome of acute pituitary apoplexy due to massive hemorrhage were reported [72, 73].

5.2. Visual disturbance

The apoplectic pituitary adenoma can expand toward the cavernous sinus, compressing the III, IV, and/or IV cranial nerves (CN), leading to various degrees of ocular palsy (diplopia and ophthalmoplegia) in 40–70% of the patients [52, 55, 74, 75].

The third CN is the most frequently affected especially when there is an abutment without invasion of the cavernous sinuses. This was explained mainly by the location of the third nerve in the same horizontal plane as the pituitary gland; pressure from lateral growth of a pituitary tumor is relatively easily transmitted to the third cranial nerve. This leads to compression of the third cranial nerve between the tumor and the interclinoid ligament, commonly resulting in the development of the third cranial nerve palsy, occurring either alone or together with damage to the other cranial nerves [52, 76].

Isolated cranial nerve palsy III in PA with direct CN III compression outside the cavernous sinus was also reported. In these cases, the tumor had some mass effect on CN III at the level of the oculomotor trigone after erosion of the posterior clinoid [77]. Multiple CN palsies and even bilateral and asymmetric lesions have been reported [78–80]. Rarely, pituitary apoplexy may present as isolated sixth cranial nerve (abducens) palsy [81].

Compression of the necrotic intrasellar mass superiorly toward the optic nerves and optic chiasma causes visual symptoms in most (75%) patients [11, 76], including decreased visual acuity; visual field defects, especially bitemporal hemianopsia; and also complete blindness and monocular blindness.

6. Differential diagnosis

As stated earlier, PA occurs in previously unknown history of pituitary mass in more than 80% of patients, the diagnosis can be challenging owing to its similarities with many other neurological conditions, and several other life-threatening conditions (**Table 3**) can lead to a delay in proper management [11].

The two most important diseases that should be considered are aneurysmal subarachnoid hemorrhage (SAH) and bacterial meningitis, subarachnoid hemorrhage [82, 83], bacterial meningitis, or parasellar abscess [84, 85].

Other differential diagnoses include subarachnoid hemorrhage, ophthalmoplegic migraine, suprasellar aneurysm, stroke and hypertensive encephalopathy, and cavernous sinus thrombosis [52, 82, 83, 85–87].

Nevertheless, a high degree of suspicion should exist in any patient presenting a severe sudden headache and visual disturbances. This aims to avoid delay in proper management.

Imaging studies are thus crucial for the diagnosis.

Differential diagnoses
Subarachnoid haemorrhage
Meningitis
Migraine
Stroke
Rathke's cleft cyst
Temporal arteritis
Tension headache
Cluster headache
Cavernous sinus thrombosis
Optic neuritis
Intracavernous carotid artery aneurysm

Table 3. Differential diagnoses of pituitary apoplexy.

7. Endocrine function

7.1. Pituitary hormone excess

As most cases of pituitary apoplexy complicate pituitary macroadenoma, many of which are secretory.

Prolactinomas are the most common (20% of cases of pituitary apoplexy); this is related to the frequency of prolactinoma in the population and to their frequent hemorrhagic nature. Hyperprolactin can also result from stalk effect [88].

It was postulated that at presentation of PA in non-PRL-secreting macroadenomas, a normal or elevated serum PRL can predict the residual anterior pituitary cell viability. Inversely a very low serum PRL level at presentation is correlated with the necrosis of the normal pituitary tissue and predicts permanent hypopituitarism [89].

More rarely PA can occur in acromegaly and Cushing's disease (too much adrenocorticotropic hormone, ACTH) in approximately 7 and 3% of cases, respectively. Co-secretion of more than one hormone may occur.

Several published series reported clinical and biochemical resolution of hormonally hyperfunctioning pituitary adenomas (including Cushing's disease and acromegaly) following pituitary apoplexy on follow-up as a result of the infarction of the pituitary tumors [90–93].

7.2. Pituitary hormone deficiency

Reviewing the series of patients with PA, one or more endocrine deficiencies can be present at the onset [22, 67, 76] and the evaluation of hormonal levels is mandatory (**Table 4**).

The pathogenesis of hypopituitarism is complex and multifactorial.

Endocrine defect
Hypopituitarism
Panhypopituitarism
ACTH deficiency
Central Hypothyroidism
Hypogonadism
Growth hormone deficiency
Diabetes insipidus
Hyponatremia

Table 4. Endocrine disorders in pituitary apoplexy.

As most episodes of PA occur in macroadenoma, the pituitary hormone deficiencies can precede the apoplectic event [22, 76].

This was explained earlier by mechanical compression of the pituitary stalk and/or the portal vessels. But more recent study suggested that it is tightly related to pressure effect of the macroadenoma, as they indicated that in patients with large pituitary adenomas, the intrasellar pressure, measured at surgery, was greater in patients who had hypopituitarism than those with intact pituitary function [94].

Moreover, the apoplexy itself can cause ischemic necrosis of the anterior pituitary secondary to a sudden rise in intrasellar pressure compressing the portal circulation, the pituitary stalk, and the pituitary gland itself [89, 95].

The most life-threatening deficit is that of adrenocorticotropic hormone (ACTH) resulting in acute central hypoadrenalism, which has been reported in more than 70% of patients [36, 52, 76]. It can result in severe hemodynamic problems. Indeed, the absence of cortisol can lead to insensitivity of the vessels to the pressor effects of endogenous or exogenous catecholamines and thus in hemodynamic instability.

Therefore, in patients with PA, empiric parental corticosteroid supplementation should be given immediately.

In the acute setting, other hormone deficiencies have less concerns. At presentation thyrotropic deficiency and gonadotropic deficiency were reported in 30–70% and 40–75% of patients, respectively [3].

Posterior pituitary involvement is not common in PA, and diabetes insipidus was reported in 3% of cases despite frequent and significant suprasellar extension in many cases [10, 96].

This may be attributable to the preservation of the posterior pituitary as a result of its different blood supply from the inferior hypophyseal artery rather than the superior hypophyseal artery that supplies the anterior pituitary and usually the tumor.

7.3. Fluid electrolyte balance: hyponatremia

Hyponatremia is a common electrolyte disturbance reported in up to 40% of patients presenting with pituitary apoplexy [22].

In most cases, hyponatremia is mostly mild, but severe hyponatremia has been reported [96–99].

It is often multifactorial and the most likely pathogenetic mechanism proposed of hyponatremia is adrenal insufficiency.

Other etiologies can include the syndrome of inappropriate ADH secretion (SIADH) resulting either from adrenal insufficiency itself or from hypothalamus irritation [99] and neurological deterioration late after initial presentation.

Hypothyroidism as common hormone deficiency in pituitary apoplexy may contribute to hyponatremia by reduction in glomerular filtration rate and elevated ADH secretion [100].

An association of a high level of atrial natriuretic peptide concomitant to a high level of ADH, a severe scenario in hyponatremic patients after pituitary apoplexy, has been demonstrated [99].

7.4. Pituitary imaging

In emergency setting, most of the patients with symptoms related to PA will undergo computed tomography (CT) as it is readily available and a rapid screening test. It is likely that, in most of them, the clinical suspicion might be something other than PA.

CT is effective in visualizing pituitary heterogeneous intrasellar and/or expansive suprasellar lesions leading to sellar enlargement (up to 94% of cases) [5, 20, 25], with a coexistence of solid and hemorrhagic areas [4, 22, 76, 101].

The CT is also able to detect subarachnoid hemorrhage and cerebral ischemia, which are the most frequent complications of PA [101].

CT is most valuable in the acute phase (up to 48 h). The recent bleeding in this phase can be missed on MRI either because of infarction or because hemorrhage is still in the form of deoxyhemoglobin. In this context, CT is able to provide an improved detection of hyperdense intralesional areas [102].

Later, during the subacute or chronic phase, in line with blood degradation, hypodense intralesional areas can be present, which increases the difficulty to make the differential diagnosis of subacute hemorrhages from other necrotic or cystic lesions (aneurysms, meningiomas, Rathke cleft cysts, germinomas, and lymphoma) [101].

This makes MRI essential to differentiate between these conditions. MRI and MR angiogram techniques also help to distinguish an aneurysm from pituitary apoplexy [4, 22, 85, 103].

Nevertheless, magnetic resonance imaging (MRI) is the radiological investigation of choice. Its findings depend on the time of onset of bleeding.

It is possible to find a fluid in the intralesional level (**Figure 1(C)**), the lower area is constituted by red cell sediment, and the cranial corresponds to free extracellular methemoglobin.

In the acute stage of pituitary apoplexy, the MRI signal is isointense or slightly hypointense on T1-weighted imaging with hypointensity on T2-weighted imaging (T2 W1). A "brushed" specific pattern of alternating subtle T1-hyperintense and T1-hypointense areas within the sellar mass may suggest apoplexy at the earlier stage [101].

Later, there is marginal signal reinforcement and the hematoma core remains isointense; in the subacute phase, the hemorrhage will appear hyperintense on T1WI as well as on T2WI. In

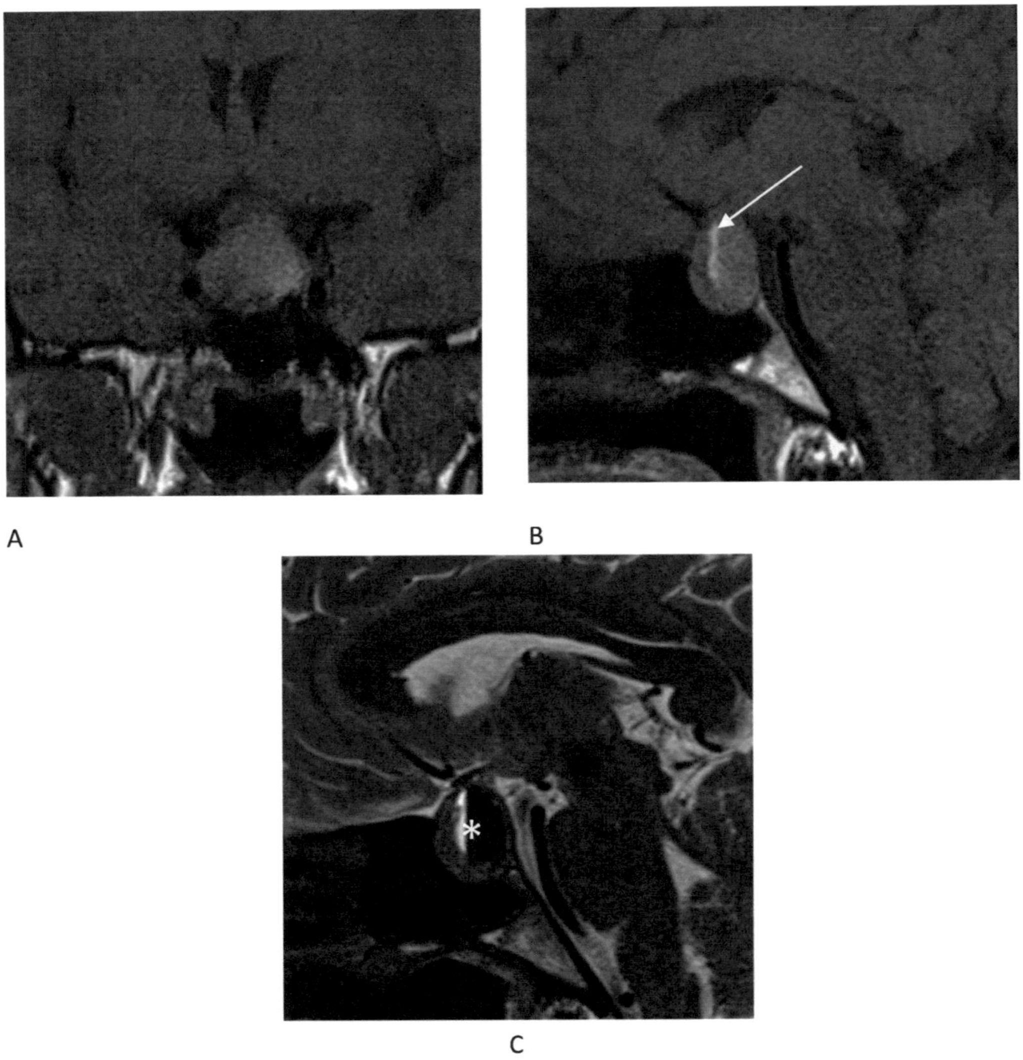

Figure 1. MRI in a pregnant patient, with symptomatic pituitary apoplexy. The lesion is globally hypointense, hemorrhagic content of the pituitary mass, and the hemorrhagic area, in T1-weighted sequences ((A) coronal section, (B) sagittal section), with a high signal intensity (arrow (B)) corresponding to the cystic area. In the same patient, the coronal T2-weighted sequences (C) showing a fluid level (asterisk) inside the pituitary lesion: the upper compartment being hyperintense while the lower is isointense.

the chronic phase, macrophages digest the clot, and the presence of hemosiderin and ferritin causes a strong hypointensity on both T1WI and T2WI [101].

In pituitary apoplexy patients, some authors reported the thickening of the sphenoid sinus mucosa related to venous engorgement in this region as an excellent sign that is present from the early stage, a reversible condition on follow-up studies that generally improves spontaneously [104]. This thickening does not indicate infectious sinusitis and thus does not rule out the surgical transsphenoidal route [103, 105].

Some published series have demonstrated the great value of special techniques as T2-weighted gradient echo to detect pituitary hemorrhage in the acute phase and chronic phase. MRI diffusion-weighted images (DWI) can be also be helpful in rare cases of ischemic pituitary necrosis without hemorrhage [105–107].

Semple et al. have demonstrated a correlation with the MRI findings and histopathology in 68% of patients with a histopathological diagnosis of hemorrhagic infarction/hemorrhage and in 82% of patients with infarction alone [103].

8. Pituitary apoplexy management

PA has long been considered as a neurosurgical emergency. However, nowadays, the conservative approach constitutes another therapeutic option in many situations. Untreated patients with apoplexy have higher morbidity and mortality. Altered consciousness, with all its associated complications, hypopituitarism, and intercurrent illnesses account for the increased morbidity and mortality of untreated patients. Although it is hard to estimate the relative increase in mortality associated without treatment, reports published before corticosteroid therapy were available indicating an approximate mortality rate of 50% [3].

The goals of treatment of PA are to improve symptoms, to decompress local structures especially the optic tract, and to avoid acute adrenal insufficiency. Hence, whether the treatment is surgical or conservative, glucocorticosteroid replacement is systematic.

8.1. Glucocorticosteroid replacement and emergency medical treatment

As corticotropic deficiency is frequently associated with pituitary apoplexy, corticosteroid should be systematically given to these patients. Thus, hydrocortisone is administered at a dose of 50 mg every 6 h [3, 108] or in the form of a 100–200 mg bolus followed by 50–100 mg every 6 h intravenously (or intramuscularly) or by 2–4 mg per hour by continuous intravenous infusion [108, 109]. Corticosteroid substitution should be associated with a careful assessment of fluid and electrolyte balance and supportive measures ensuring hemodynamic stability. Once glucocorticoids are administered, clinical improvement is invariably observed, and hemodynamic stability becomes easier to maintain. The glucocorticoids are administered in supraphysiological doses to serve not only as replacement for endogenous hormone deficiency but also to help control the effect of edema on parasellar structures [3].

8.2. Neurosurgical treatment

8.2.1. Technique

If surgical management is chosen, the transsphenoidal approach is almost always recommended, because it allows good decompression of the optic pathways and neuroanatomic structures in contact with the tumor and because it is associated with low postoperative morbidity and mortality [11]. Usually, necroticohemorrhagic material is evacuated as soon as the incision of the tumor capsule is made. The purpose of the surgery is the decompression of the optical pathways; the surgeon should try to identify the sellar diaphragm. In case of invasive pituitary adenoma, a maximum but incomplete resection is ensured by taking all the precautions to avoid damaging the cranial nerves or the carotids in case of invasion of the cavernous sinuses.

8.2.2. Timing

The timing of pituitary surgery is controversial, as no randomized trials comparing different strategies with strong evidence have been performed. However, most studies indicate that surgical treatment, usually within 7 days after the apoplectic event, leads to higher rates of visual impairment recovery [11, 110].

Occasionally, patients are clinically or biochemically hypothyroid at presentation. Unless the hypothyroidism is severe, the surgical decompression needs not be delayed, provided the anesthesiologists and the management team are aware of the patient's condition to avoid medications and procedures that are particularly deleterious and that can potentially worsen clinical symptoms [3].

8.2.3. Outcomes

Surgical decompression normalizes visual acuity in about one-half of cases and improves it in another 6–36% of cases [52, 53]. Visual field defects normalize after surgery in 30–60% of cases and improve in another 50%. Ocular motility dysfunction can resolve spontaneously, with or without surgery [111].

Pituitary deficiencies are usually not expected to recover [19, 112]. In addition, it seems that apoplexy worsens endocrine outcome: hormonal prognosis after elective pituitary surgery is poorer in patients with PA than in patients without PA [9]. This is explained mainly by the damage to the normal gland from the initial apoplectic event. Another important point is that, in this acute setting, the operation may be performed by an on-call neurosurgeon rather than by a skilled pituitary neurosurgeon, as underlined in UK guidelines [11], and this may increase the risk of adverse events.

For tumoral outcome, *c*omplete tumor removal is reported in 48–66% of patients and subtotal resection in 23–52% of patients [95]. Tumor recurrence has been described in 6–11% of patients [112].

8.2.4. Surgical complications

Surgery may also be harmful, with a risk of postoperative cerebrospinal fluid leakage, permanent diabetes insipidus caused by posterior pituitary damage, meningitis, and an increased likelihood of hypopituitarism due to removal or damage to normal pituitary tissue. Fortunately, in experienced pituitary centers, these complications are very rare [5].

8.3. Conservative approach: rationale, modalities, and outcomes

Several reports have documented that spontaneous neurological recovery is possible despite unilateral ophthalmoplegia and partial visual field defects, which has suggested that nonoperative medical management of patients with PA may be appropriate in many situations.

In 1995, Maccagnan et al. reported the results of a prospective study in which they treated PA with high-dose steroids (2 to 16 mg of dexamethasone daily). Only patients whose visual impairment or altered consciousness failed to improve underwent surgery. Conservative treatment was possible on 7 of 12 patients, and only 5 patients had needed surgery. Visual deficits regress in 6 of the 7 patients and improved in the remaining patients. The posttreatment prevalence of pituitary hormone deficiency and the incidence of tumor regrowth were similar in conservatively and surgically treated patients [113].

Thus, conservative therapy involved supportive therapy, continued use of supraphysiological doses of glucocorticoids for several weeks, and hormone replacement therapy. Improvement in neurological symptoms is often seen in the majority of patients treated conservatively, at times to a similar degree to that seen in surgically treated patients. However, worsening of pituitary function is usually seen in many of these patients [114]. For functioning pituitary adenomas, hormonal secretion must be also evaluated: hormonal levels could be low, be normal, or remain high after apoplexy [11]. For tumoral outcomes, additional treatment is not necessary in most cases, as tumors usually diminish and even disappear without surgical intervention [10]. It seems that a single large hypodense area within the tumor on CT might be associated with better subsequent tumor shrinkage than are several small hypodense areas [113].

8.4. Surgical or conservative treatment?

PA is characterized by a highly capricious course, and randomized prospective studies with strong evidence about this syndrome are lacking, which makes optimal management of acute PA controversial. Although guidelines, as the one from the UK, proposed an algorithm for PA management, randomized trials comparing both strategies are needed for strong evidence [11, 112]. Hence, the decision of surgical treatment or conservative management should be individualized and made by experts from a multidisciplinary team including endocrinologists, neurologists, ophthalmologists, and neurosurgeon [11].

The risk-benefit ratio of conservative treatment versus surgery must be carefully evaluated, in terms of visual outcome, pituitary function and also subsequent tumor growth. On the other hand, the potentially serious complications of surgery need to be taken into consideration [115].

8.4.1. Background

In spite of the methodological limits of the studies available on this subject, these data have constituted the rationale guiding the therapeutic choice of PA.

The outcome of visual acuity, field defect, or ophthalmoplegia is similar with surgery or conservative treatment. Unfortunately, visual outcome is poorer in patients with more severe disorders such as monocular or binocular blindness, irrespective of whether management is conservative or surgical [56, 116, 117]. It has been argued that conservatively treated patients may have less severe visual defects than surgically treated patients and that this might explain why the improvement is at least as good in the former as in the latter [3, 11, 118]. The number of patients with visual defects was effectively higher in the surgical groups of published series [53, 76].

For endocrine prognosis, whatever the management approach, the hormonal outcome is poor in patients with PA, who frequently suffer irreversible pituitary damage [11].

Concerning the outcome of the pituitary tumor, very few studies have compared the degree of tumor disappearance between patients receiving surgery and conservative treatment for apoplexy. The reported results were very different: the incidence of recurrence was similar between the two approaches in one study [76], higher after surgery in one other [56], and lower after surgery in two others [52]. Thus, the optimal approach for tumor control is difficult to judge. Whatever the therapeutic choice in the acute event, additional forms of therapy can be used to control residual tumor growth, depending on the type of tumor, including a dopamine agonist for documented prolactinomas or a somatostatin analogue for documented growth hormone-secreting tumors. Gamma Knife stereotactic radiosurgery can also be used on these patients and on patients with nonsecreting adenomas [3].

8.4.2. MRI's contribution to the therapeutic choice

MRI did not predict the severity of ocular paresis or field defects. The size of the tumor on MRI is not actually a strong argument for therapeutic choice. Even when the tumor was very large, conservative management was accompanied by tumor shrinkage [76]. However, some MRI findings were found to be associated with clinical status and outcome: patients with simple infarction had less severe clinical features and better outcomes than those with hemorrhagic infarction or hemorrhage [70].

All these data from the literature have allowed deducing overall the place of, respectively, the conservative approach and the surgical treatment in the management of PA.

8.4.3. Surgical treatment indications

According to the majority of authors, surgical intervention should be considered in patients with severely reduced visual acuity, severe and persistent visual field defects, and deteriorating level of consciousness despite glucocorticoid replacement and hydroelectrolytic support [109]. Ocular paresis because of involvement of III, IV, or VI cranial nerves in the cavernous sinus is not in itself an indication for immediate surgery. Resolution will typically occur within days or weeks with conservative management [11].

The UK Guidelines for PA recommend a scoring system (**Table 5**), calculated using visual acuity, visual defects, cranial nerve palsies, and the Glasgow Coma Scale. The PA score ranges from 0 to 10, and surgery usually is indicated for scores ≥4 [11]. Another scoring system, from the Massachusetts General Hospital, proposes grading patients on a scale from 1 to 5: grade 1 for asymptomatic individuals, grade 2 for patients with symptoms due to endocrinopathy, grade 3 for patients with headache, grade 4 for patients with ocular paresis, and grade 5 for patients with visual deficits or a low Glasgow Coma Scale score. Patients with grade 5 should be submitted to surgery [59].

8.4.4. Conservative management indications

For conservative approach, it is safe in patients with pituitary tumor apoplexy who are without any neuro-ophthalmic signs or mild and stable signs or those with evidence of early improvement after administration of glucocorticoids [76]. This would be particularly

Variable	Points
Level of consciousness	
Glasgow coma scale 15	0
Glasgow coma scale 8–14	2
Glasgow coma scale _8	4
Visual acuity	
Normal 10/10 (or no change from pre-PA visual acuity)	0
Reduced, unilateral	1
Reduced, bilateral	2
Visual field defects	
Normal	0
Unilateral defect	1
Bilateral defect	2
Ocular paresis	
Absent	0
Present – Unilateral	1
Bilateral	2

[From S. Rajasekaran et al: UK guidelines for the management of pituitary apoplexy.*[11]* with permission.

Table 5. Pituitary apoplexy score (PAS).

applicable in patients with prolactin-secreting adenomas, with whom dopamine agonists are very effective not only in controlling hyperprolactinemia but also in reducing the size of the adenoma [3]. "Wait-and-see" approach should be also considered in patients with significant clinical comorbidities.

If conservative treatment is chosen, then careful monitoring of visual signs and symptoms is necessary, and surgical decompression is recommended if visual disorders do not improve or if they deteriorate [5, 11, 59].

8.5. Follow-up

All patients with pituitary apoplexy need follow-up by endocrine and neurosurgical teams. They require repeated assessment of pituitary and visual function (visual acuity, eye movements, and visual fields), at 4–6 weeks. Thereafter, hormonal reevaluation must be performed every 6–12 months to determine whether or not the pituitary defect is permanent and the possible hypersecretory nature of the adenoma and to optimize hormonal replacement [109].

Sellar MRI should be repeated in 3–6 months, annually for 5 years, and biannually after that to monitor tumor progression/recurrence [119]. The presence of an "empty sella" is often observed [117].

Morbidity and mortality in patients with pituitary tumor apoplexy have declined in the past six decades. Four factors may have contributed to the improved survival: improved diagnostic accuracy, use of glucocorticoids, use of more sophisticated supportive therapy, and refinements in surgical techniques and postoperative care [3]. Currently, mortality in the acute setting is less than 2% [120].

9. Conclusion

PA is uncommon but a potentially life-threatening complication due to acute infarction or hemorrhage within a preexisting pituitary adenoma. Its pathophysiology, including extrinsic compression of arterial supply or intrinsic tumoral factors, is still controversial. In terms of triggering factors, the most common include major surgery. The classical presentation is highly suspected when an acute lancinating headache is combined with visual disturbance, cranial nerve palsy, and hypopituitarism. MRI is a fundamental step to evaluate the pituitary infarct and hemorrhage and to rule out other pathologies. For the management of PA, corticosteroids should be systematically administered. However, the therapeutic choice between surgery and conservative treatment is controversial and should be made by experts from a multidisciplinary team. The surgical management which used to be considered as the first-line treatment of this acute condition is now reserved for patients with severe neuro-ophthalmic signs. Improvement of the diagnostic means and the therapeutic management has allowed a better PA prognosis which is preserved in most of the cases. Reevaluation of the pituitary function and tumor mass is mandatory in the months after the acute apoplectic episode to adjust hormonal substitution, to detect the possible hypersecretory nature of the adenoma, and to initiate follow-up of a possible tumor remnant.

Author details

Manel Jemel[1]*, Wafa Alaya[2], Fedia Boubaker[2], Olfa Berrich[2] and Baha Zantour[2]

*Address all correspondence to: maneljemel@gmail.com

1 Department of Endocrinology, National Institute of Nutrition and Food Technology, Tunis, Tunisia

2 Department of Endocrinology and Internal Medicine, University Hospital Taher Sfar, Mahdia, Tunisia

References

[1] Bailey P. Pathological report of a case of acromegaly, with special reference to the lesion in the hypophysis cerebri and in the thyroid gland; and a case of haemorrhage into the pituitary. The Philadelphia medical Journal. 1898;**1**:789-792

[2] Brougham M, Heusner AP, Adams RD. Acute degenerative changes in adenomas of the pituitary body-with special reference to pituitary apoplexy. Journal of Neurosurgery. 1950;**7**:421-439

[3] Nawar RN, Abdel Mannan D, Selman WR, Arafah BM. Pituitary tumor apoplexy: A review. Journal of Intensive Care Medicine. 2008;**23**:75-90. DOI: 10.1177/0885066607312992

[4] Dubuisson AS, Beckers A, Stevenaert A. Classical pituitary tumour apoplexy: Clinical features, management and outcomes in a series of 24 patients. Clinical Neurology and Neurosurgery. 2007;**109**:63-70. DOI: 10.1016/j.clineuro.2006.01.006

[5] Fernandez A, Karavitaki N, Wass JA. Prevalence of pituitary adenomas: A community-based, cross-sectional study in Banbury (Oxfordshire, UK). Clinical Endocrinology. 2010;**72**:377-382. DOI: 10.1111/j.1365-2265.2009.03667.x

[6] Raappana A, Koivukangas J, Ebeling T, Pirilä T. Incidence of pituitary adenomas in northern Finland in 1992-2007. The Journal of Clinical Endocrinology and Metabolism. 2010;**95**:4268-4275. DOI: 10.1210/jc.2010-0537

[7] Briet C, Salenave S, Bonneville JF, Laws ER, Chanson P. Pituitary apoplexy. Endocrine Reviews. 2015;**36**:622-645. DOI: 10.1210/er.2015-1042

[8] Nielsen EH, Lindholm J, Bjerre P, et al. Frequent occurrence of pituitary apoplexy in patients with nonfunctioning pituitary adenoma. Clinical Endocrinology. 2006;**64**: 319-322. DOI: 10.1111/j.1365-2265.2006.02463.x

[9] Wildemberg LE, Glezer A, Bronstein MD, Gadelha MR. Apoplexy in nonfunctioning pituitary adenomas. Pituitary. 2018;**21**:138-144. DOI: 10.1007/s11102-018-0870-x

[10] Möller-Goede DL, Brändle M, Landau K, Bernays RL, Schmid C. Pituitary apoplexy: Re-evaluation of risk factors for bleeding into pituitary adenomas and impact on outcome. European Journal of Endocrinology. 2011;**164**:37-43. DOI: 10.1530/EJE-10-0651

[11] Rajasekaran S, Vanderpump M, Baldeweg S, et al. UK guidelines for the management of pituitary apoplexy. Clinical Endocrinology (Oxford). 2011;**74**:9-20. DOI: 10.1111/j.1365-2265.2010.03913.x

[12] Vargas G, Gonzalez B, Ramirez C, Ferreira A, Espinosa E, Mendoza V, Guinto G, Lopez-Felix B, Zepeda E, Mercado M. Clinical characteristics and treatment outcome of 485 patients with nonfunctioning pituitary macroadenomas. International Journal of Endocrinology. 2015:756069. DOI: 10.1155/2015/756069

[13] Jankoswski PP, Crawford JR, Khanna P, Malicki DM, Ciacci JD, Levy ML. Pituitary tumor apoplexy in adolescents. World Neurosurgery. 2015;**83**:644-645. DOI: 10.1016/j.wneu.2014.12.026

[14] Glezer A, Bronstein MD. Pituitary apoplexy: Pathophysiology, diagnosis and management. The Archives of Endocrinology and Metabolism. 2015;**59**:259-264. DOI: 10.1590/2359-3997000000047

[15] Semple PL, De Villiers JC, Bowen RM, Lopes MB, Laws ER. Pituitary apoplexy: Do histological features influence the clinical presentation and outcome? Journal of Neurosurgery. 2006;**104**:931-937. DOI: 10.3171/jns.2006.104.6.931

[16] Sarwar KN, Huda MS, Van de Velde V, Hopkins L, Luck S, Preston R, et al. The prevalence and natural history of pituitary hemorrhage in prolactinoma. The Journal of Clinical Endocrinology and Metabolism. 2013;**98**(6):2362-2367. DOI: 10.1210/jc.2013-1249

[17] Oldfield EH, Merrill MJ. Apoplexy of pituitary adenomas: The perfect storm. Journal of Neurosurgery. 2015;**122**:1444-1449. DOI: 10.3171/2014.10.JNS141720

[18] Turner HE, Nagy Z, Gatter KC, Esiri MM, Harris AL, Wass JA. Angiogenesis in pituitary adenomas and the normal pituitary gland. The Journal of Clinical Endocrinology and Metabolism. 2000;**85**:1159-1162. DOI: 10.1210/jcem.85.3.6485

[19] Bills DC, Meyer FB, Laws ER Jr, et al. A retrospective analysis of pituitary apoplexy. Neurosurgery. 1993;**33**:602-609

[20] Kruse A, Astrup J, Cold GE, Hansen HH. Pressure and blood flow in pituitary adenomas measured during transsphenoidal surgery. British Journal of Neurosurgery. 1992;**6**:333-341

[21] Xekouki P, Mastroyiannis SA, Avgeropoulos D, et al. Familial pituitary apoplexy as the only presentation of a novel AIP mutation. Endocrine-Related Cancer. 2013;**20**:5. DOI: 10.1530/ERC-13-0218

[22] Louwerens M, de Herder WW, Postema PT, Tanghe HL, Lamberts SW. Pituitary insufficiency and regression of acromegaly caused by pituitary apoplexy following cerebral angiography. European Journal of Endocrinology. 1996;**134**:737-740. DOI: 10.1530/eje.0.1340737

[23] Skljarevski V, Khoshyomn S, Fries TJ. Pituitary apoplexy in the setting of coronary angiography. Journal of Neuroimaging. 2003;**13**:276-279. DOI: 10.1177/1051228403254656

[24] Weisberg LA. Pituitary apoplexy. Association of degenerative change in pituitary adenoma with radiotherapy and detection by cerebral computed tomography. The American Journal of Medicine. 1977;**63**:109-115. DOI: 10.1016/0002-9343(77)90122-X

[25] Bhatt G, Bhatt AD, Silverman CL, Dragun AE. Pituitary apoplexy after hypo-fractionated stereotactic radiotherapy. Journal of Solid Tumors; 26 Mar 2013;**3**(3):22

[26] Smidt MH, van der Vliet A, Wesseling P, de Vries J, Twickler TB, Vos PE. Pituitary apoplexy after mild head injury misinterpreted as bacterial meningitis. European Journal of Neurology. 2007;**14**:e7-e8. DOI: 10.1111/j.1468-1331.2007.01644.x

[27] Mayrin JV, Laufgraben M. Pituitary apoplexy following cardiac surgery: A case report and review of the literature. Endocrinologist. 2007;**7**(4):214-216. DOI: 10.1097/TEN.0b013e3180ca7786

[28] Liberale G, Bruninx G, Vanderkelen B, Dubois E, Vandueren E, Verhelst G. Pituitary apoplexy after aortic abdominal aneurysm surgery: A case report. Acta Chirurgica Belgica. 2006;**106**:77-80. DOI: 10.1080/00015458.2006.11679839

[29] Mizuno T. Pituitary apoplexy with third cranial nerve palsy after off-pump coronary artery bypasses grafting. Interactive CardioVascular and Thoracic Surgery. 2011;**13**:240-242. DOI: 10.1510/icvts.2011.268854

[30] Levy E, Korach A, Merin G, Feinsod M, Glenville B. Pituitary apoplexy and CABG: Should we change our strategy? The Annals of Thoracic Surgery. 2007;**84**:1388-1390. DOI: 10.1016/j.athoracsur.2007.05.017

[31] Randeva HS, Schoebel J, Byrne J, Esiri M, Adams CB, Wass JA. Classical pituitary apoplexy: Clinical features, management and outcome. Clinical Endocrinology. 1999;**51**:181-188. DOI: 10.1046/j.1365-2265.1999.00754.x

[32] Mou C, Han T, Zhao H, Wang S, Qu Y. Clinical features and immunohistochemical changes of pituitary apoplexy. Journal of Clinical Neuroscience. 2009;**16**:64-68. DOI: 10.1016/j.jocn.2008.02.012

[33] Biousse V, Newman NJ, Oyesiku NM. Precipitating factors in pituitary apoplexy. Neurology, Neurosurgery & Psychiatry. 2001;**71**:542-545. DOI: 10.1136/jnnp.71.4.542

[34] Rotman-Pikielny P, Patronas N, Papanicolaou DA. Pituitary apoplexy induced by corticotrophin releasing hormone in a patient with Cushing's disease. Clinical Endocrinology. 2003;**58**:545-549. DOI: 10.1046/j.1365-2265.2003.01720.x

[35] Yamamoto T, Yano S, Kuroda J-i, Yu H, Hide T, Kuratsu J-i. Pituitary apoplexy associated with endocrine stimulation test: Endocrine stimulation test, treatment, and outcome. Research article. Case Reports in Endocrinology. 2012. https://doi.org/10.1155/2012/826901

[36] Semple PL, Jane JA Jr, Laws ER Jr. Clinical relevance of precipitating factors in pituitary apoplexy. Neurosurgery. 2007;**61**:956-961. discussion 961-962. DOI: 10.1227/01.neu.0000303191.57178.2a

[37] Heide LJ, van Tol KM, Doorenbos B. Pituitary apoplexy presenting during pregnancy. The Netherlands Journal of Medicine. 2004;**62**:393-396. http://www.njmonline.nl/getpdf.php?id=259

[38] Parihar V, Yadav YR, Sharma D. Pituitary apoplexy in a pregnant woman. Annals of Indian Academy of Neurology. 2009;**12**:54-55. DOI: 10.4103/0972-2327.48861

[39] Keane F, Egan AM, Navin P, Brett F, Dennedy MC. Gonadotropin-releasing hormone agonist-induced pituitary apoplexy. Endocrinology, Diabetes & Metabolism Case Reports. 2016;**2016**:160021. DOI: 10.1530/EDM-16-0021

[40] Massoud W, Paparel P, Lopez JG, Perrin P, Daumont M, Ruffion A. Discovery of a pituitary adenoma following a gonadotropin-releasing hormone agonist in a patient with prostate cancer. International Journal of Urology. 2006;**13**:303-304. DOI: 10.1111/j.1442-2042.2006.01237.x

[41] Huang TY, Lin JP, Lieu AS, Chen YT, Chen HS, Jang MY, Shen JT, Wu WJ, Huang SP, Juan YS. Pituitary apoplexy induced by gonadotropin-releasing hormone agonists for treating prostate cancer-report of first Asian case. World Journal of Surgical Oncology. 2013;**11**:254. https://www.ncbi.nlm.nih.gov/pmc/articles/PMC3851712/

[42] Knoepfelmacher M, Gomes MC, Melo ME, Mendonça BB. Pituitary apoplexy during therapy with cabergoline in an adolescent male with prolactin-secreting macroadenoma. Pituitary. 2004;**7**:83-87. DOI: 10.1186/1477-7819-11-254

[43] Balarini Lima GA, Machado Ede O, Dos Santos Silva CM, Filho PN, Gadelha MR. Pituitary apoplexy during treatment of cystic macroprolactinomas with cabergoline. Pituitary. 2008;**11**:287-292. DOI: 10.1007/s11102-007-0046-6

[44] Colao A, Di Sarno A, Landi ML, Scavuzzo F, Cappabianca P, Pivonello R, Volpe R, Di Salle F, Cirillo S, Annunziato L, Lombardi G. Macroprolactinoma shrinkage during cabergoline treatment is greater in naïve patients than in patients pretreated with other dopamine agonists: A prospective study in 110 patients. The Journal of Clinical Endocrinology and Metabolism. 2000;**85**:2247-2252. DOI: 10.1210/jcem.85.6.6657

[45] Vroonen L, Jaffrain-Rea ML, Petrossians P, Tamagno G, Chanson P, Vilar L, Borson-Chazot F, Naves LA, Brue T, Gatta B, Delemer B, Ciccarelli E, Beck-Peccoz P, Caron P,

Daly AF, Beckers A. Prolactinomas resistant to standard doses of cabergoline: A multicenter study of 92 patients. European Journal of Endocrinology. 2012;**167**:651-662. DOI: 10.1530/EJE-12-0236

[46] Delgrange E, Daems T, Verhelst J, Abs R, Maiter D. Characterization of resistance to the prolactin-lowering effects of cabergoline in macroprolactinomas: A study in 122 patients. European Journal of Endocrinology. 2009;**160**:747-752. DOI: 10.1530/EJE-09-0012

[47] Nagarajan DV, Bird D, Papouchado M. Pituitary apoplexy following anticoagulation for acute coronary syndrome. Heart. 2003;**89**:10. DOI: 10.1136/heart.89.1.10

[48] Uemura MMF, Shimomura R, Fujinami J, Toyoda K. Pituitary apoplexy during treatment with dabigatran. Neurology and Clinical Neuroscience. 2013;**1**:82-83. DOI: 10.1002/ncn3.18

[49] Doglietto F, Costi E, Villaret AB, Mardighian D, Fontanella MM, Giustina A. New oral anticoagulants and pituitary apoplexy. Pituitary. 2016;**19**(2):232-234. DOI: 10.1007/s11102-014-0616-3

[50] Maïza JC, Bennet A, Thorn-Kany M, Lagarrigue J, Caron P. Pituitary apoplexy and idiopathic thrombocytopenic purpura: A new case and review of the literature. Pituitary. 2004;**7**:189-192. DOI: 10.1007/s11102-005-1760-6

[51] Wongpraparut N, Pleanboonlers N, Suwattee P, Rerkpattanapipat P, Turtz A, Moster M, Gala I, Kim YN. Pituitary apoplexy in a patient with acute myeloid leukemia and thrombocytopenia. Pituitary. 2000;**3**:113-116. DOI: 10.1023/A:1009909908942

[52] Sibal L, Ball SG, Connolly V, James RA, Kane P, Kelly WF, Kendall-Taylor P, Mathias D, Perros P, Quinton R, Vaidya B. Pituitary apoplexy: A review of clinical presentation, management and outcome in 45 cases. Pituitary. 2004;**7**:157-163. DOI: 10.1007/s11102-005-1050-3

[53] Leyer C, Castinetti F, Morange I, Gueydan M, Oliver C, Conte-Devolx B, Dufour H, Brue T. A conservative management is preferable in milder forms of pituitary tumor apoplexy. Journal of Endocrinological Investigation. 2011;**34**:502-509. DOI: 10.3275/7241

[54] Vargas G, Gonzalez B, Guinto G, Mendoza V, López-Félix B, Zepeda E, Mercado M. Pituitary apoplexy in nonfunctioning pituitary macroadenomas: A case-control study. Endocrine Practice. 2014;**20**:1274-1280. DOI: 10.4158/EP14120.OR

[55] Pal A, Capatina C, Tenreiro AP, Guardiola PD, Byrne JV, Cudlip S, Karavitaki N, Wass JA. Pituitary apoplexy in non-functioning pituitary adenomas: Long term follow up is important because of significant numbers of tumour recurrences. Clinical Endocrinology. 2011;**75**:501-504. DOI: 10.1111/j.1365-2265.2011.04068.x

[56] Gruber A, Clayton J, Kumar S, Robertson I, Howlett TA, Mansell P. Pituitary apoplexy: Retrospective review of 30 patients–is surgical intervention always necessary? British Journal of Neurosurgery. 2006;**20**:379-385. DOI: 10.1080/02688690601046678

[57] Semple PL, Webb MK, de Villiers JC, Laws ER Jr. Pituitary apoplexy. Neurosurgery. 2005;**56**:65-73. discussion 62-73. DOI: 10.1227/01.NEU.0000144840.55247.38

[58] Khaldi M, Ben Hamouda K, Jemel H, Kallel J, Zemmel I. Pituitary apoplexy. Report of 25 patients. Neuro-Chirurgie. 2006;**52**:330-338. DOI: NCHIR-09-2006-52-4-0028-3770-1010 19-200604684

[59] Jho DH, Biller BM, Agarwalla PK, Swearingen B. Pituitary apoplexy: Large surgical series with grading system. World Neurosurgery. 2014;**82**:781-790. DOI: 10.1016/j.wneu.2014.06.005

[60] Chan D, Rong TC, Dalan R. Cushing's disease presenting with pituitary apoplexy. Journal of Clinical Neuroscience. 2012;**19**:1586-1589. DOI: 10.1016/j.jocn.2011.10.017

[61] Kinoshita Y, Tominaga A, Usui S, Arita K, Sugiyama K, Kurisu K. Impact of subclinical haemorrhage on the pituitary gland in patients with pituitary adenomas. Clinical Endocrinology. 2014;**80**:720-725. DOI: 10.1111/cen.12349

[62] Scheithauer BW, Jaap AJ, Horvath E, Kovacs K, Lloyd RV, Meyer FB, Laws ER Jr, Young WF Jr. Clinically silent corticotroph tumors of the pituitary gland. Neurosurgery. 2000;**47**:723-729. discussion 729-730. DOI: 10.1097/00006123-200009000-00039

[63] Sahli R, Christ ER, Seiler R, Kappeler A, Vajtai I. Clinicopathologic correlations of silent corticotroph adenomas of the pituitary: Report of four cases and literature review. Pathology, Research and Practice. 2006;**202**:457-464. DOI: 10.1016/j.prp.2006.01.007

[64] Lubina A, Olchovsky D, Berezin M, Ram Z, Hadani M, Shimon I. Management of pituitary apoplexy: Clinical experience with 40 patients. Acta Neurochirurgica. 2005;**147**:151-157. DOI: 10.1007/s00701-004-0413-2

[65] Russel SJ, Miller KK. Pituitary apoplexy. In: Swearingen B, Biller BMK, editors. Diagnosis and Management of Pituitary Disorders. Totowa, NJ: Humana Press; 2008. pp. 353-375

[66] Shimon I. Clinical features of pituitary apoplexy. In: Turgut M, Mahapatra AK, Powell M, Muthukumar N, editors. Pituitary Apoplexy. Berlin, Heidelberg: Springer-Verlag; 2014. pp. 49-54

[67] Johnston PC, Hamrahian AH, Weil RJ, Kennedy L. Pituitary tumor apoplexy. Journal of Clinical Neuroscience. 2015;**22**(6):939-944. DOI: 10.1016/j.jocn.2014.11.023

[68] Satyarthee GD, Mahapatra AK. Pituitary apoplexy in a child presenting with massive subarachnoid and intraventricular hemorrhage. Journal of Clinical Neuroscience. 2005;**12**:94-96. DOI: 10.1016/j.jocn.2003.10.030

[69] Sugand K, Metcalfe D, Jaiganesh T. Subarachnoid haemorrhage with pituitary adenoma. In: Turgut M, Mahapatra AK, Powell M, Muthukumar N, editors. Pituitary Apoplexy. Berlin, Heidelberg, Germany: Springer-Verlag; 2014. pp. 55-67

[70] Ahmed SK, Semple PL. Cerebral ischaemia in pituitary apoplexy. Acta Neurochirurgica. 2008;**150**:1193-1196. discussion 1196. DOI: 10.1007/s00701-008-0130-3

[71] Verma R, Singh S, Patil TB. Thalamic infarction in pituitary apoplexy syndrome. BML Case Reports. 2012 Oct;**12**:2012. DOI: 10.1136/bcr-2012-006993

[72] Bauer M, Lang C, Patzelt D. Sudden death due to pituitary apoplexy. Legal Medicine (Tokyo). 2001;**3**(3):183-186. DOI: 10.1016/S1344-6223(01)00026-8

[73] Shields LB, Balko MG, Hunsaker JC 3rd. Sudden and unexpected death from pituitary tumor apoplexy. Journal of Forensic Sciences. 2012;**57**:262-266. DOI: 10.1111/j.1556-4029.2011.01906.x

[74] Hage R, Eshraghi SR, Oyesiku NM, Ioachimescu AG, Newman NJ, Biousse V, Bruce BB. Third, fourth, and sixth cranial nerve palsies in pituitary apoplexy. World Neurosurgery. 2016;**94**:447-452. DOI: 10.1016/j.wneu.2016.07.026

[75] Zhu X, Wang Y, Zhao X, Jiang C, Zhang Q, Jiang W, Chen H, Shou X, Zhao Y, Li Y, Li S, Ye H. Incidence of pituitary apoplexy and its risk factors in chinese people: A database study of patients with pituitary adenoma. PLoS One. 2015;**10**:e0139088. DOI: 10.1371/journal.pone.0139088

[76] Ayuk J, McGregor EJ, Mitchell RD, Gittoes NJ. Acute management of pituitary apoplexy–surgery or conservative management? Clinical Endocrinology. 2004;**61**:747-752. DOI: 10.1111/j.1365-2265.2004.02162.x

[77] Kobayashi H, Kawabori M, Terasaka S, Murata J, Houkin K. A possible mechanism of isolated oculomotor nerve palsy by apoplexy of pituitary adenoma without cavernous sinus invasion: A report of two cases. Acta Neurochirurgica. 2011;**153**(12):2453-2456. DOI: 10.1007/s00701-011-1165-4

[78] Delgado-Alvarado M, Riancho J, Riancho-Zarrabeitia L, Sedano MJ, Polo JM, Berciano J. Unilateral total ophthalmoplegia without visual loss as the presenting form of a pituitary apoplexy. Revista Clínica Española. 2013;**213**:e67-e70. DOI: 10.1016/j.rce.2013.05.009

[79] Diyora B, Nayak N, Kukreja S, Kamble H. Sudden onset isolated complete third nerve palsy due to pituitary apoplexy. Oman Journal of Ophthalmology. 2011;**4**:32-34. DOI: 10.4103/0974-620X.77661

[80] Tanriverdi F, Karaca Z, Oner A, Durak AC, Selcuklu A, Unluhizarci K, Kelestimur F. Complete surgical resolution of bilateral total opthalmoplegia without visual field defect in an acromegalic patient presented with pituitary apoplexy. Endocrine Journal. 2007;**54**:681-684. DOI: 10.1507/endocrj.K07-008

[81] Zoli M, Mazzatenta D, Pasquini E, Ambrosetto P, Frank G. Cavernous sinus apoplexy presenting isolated sixth cranial nerve palsy: Case report. Pituitary. 2012;**15**(Suppl 1):37-40. DOI: 10.1007/s11102-011-0312-5

[82] Tedd HM, Tuckett J, Arun C, Dhar A. An unusual case of sudden onset headache due to pituitary apoplexy: A case report and review of the new UK guidelines. The Journal of the Royal College of Physicians of Edinburgh. 2012;**42**:119-123. DOI: 10.4997/JRCPE.2012.206

[83] Ni CD, Lambert J. Sudden headache, third nerve palsy and visual deficit: Thinking outside the subarachnoid haemorrhage box. Age and Ageing. 2013;**42**:810-812. DOI: 10.1093/ageing/aft088

[84] Wong SH, Das K, Javadpour M. Pituitary apoplexy initially mistaken for bacterial meningitis. BMJ Case Reports. 5 Sept 2013;**2013**:bcr2013009223

[85] Paisley AN, Syed AA. Pituitary apoplexy masquerading as bacterial meningitis. Canadian Medical Association Journal. 2012;**184**:1812. DOI: 10.1503/cmaj.120174

[86] Silvestrini M, Matteis M, Cupini LM, Troisi E, Bernardi G, Floris R. Ophthalmoplegic migraine-like syndrome due to pituitary apoplexy. Headache. 1994;**34**:484-486. DOI: 10.1111/j.1526-4610.1994. hed3408484.x

[87] Verrees M, Arafah BM, Selman WR. Pituitary tumor apoplexy: Characteristics, treatment, and outcomes. Neurosurgical Focus. 2004;**16**:E6. DOI: 10.3171/foc.2004.16.4.7

[88] Skinner DC. Rethinking the stalk effect: A new hypothesis explaining suprasellar tumor-induced hyperprolactinemia. Medical Hypotheses. 2009;**72**(3):309-310. DOI: 10.1016/j.mehy.2008.08.030

[89] Zayour DH, Selman WR, Arafah BM. Extreme elevation of intrasellar pressure in patients with pituitary tumor apoplexy: Relation to pituitary function. The Journal of Clinical Endocrinology and Metabolism. 2004;**89**:5649-5654. DOI: 10.1210/jc.2004-0884

[90] Marko NF, Hamrahian AH, Hatipoglu B, et al. Relapsing remitting hypercortisolism in Cushing's disease due to intratumoral hemorrhages in pituitary microadenoma. Journal of Clinical Neuroscience. 2013;**20**:753-756. DOI: 10.1016/j.jocn.2012.05.039

[91] Cinar N, Metin Y, Dagdelen S, et al. Spontaneous remission of acromegaly after infarctive apoplexy with a possible relation to MRI and diabetes mellitus. Neuro Endocrinology Letters. 2013;**34**:339-342. DOI: 10.1210/endo-meetings. 2010.PART3.P6.P3-283

[92] Fraser LA, Lee D, Cooper P, et al. Remission of acromegaly after pituitary apoplexy: Case report and review of literature. Endocrine Practice. 2009;**15**:725-731. DOI: 10.4158/EP09126.CR

[93] Choudhry OJ, Choudhry AJ, Nunez EA, et al. Pituitary tumor apoplexy in patients with Cushing's disease: Endocrinologic and visual outcomes after transsphenoidal surgery. Pituitary. 2012;**15**:428-435. DOI: 10.1007/s11102-011-0342-z

[94] Arafah BM, Prunty D, Ybarra J, Hlavin ML, Selman WR. The dominant role of increased intrasellar pressure in the pathogenesis of hypopituitarism, hyperprolactinemia, and headaches in patients with pituitary adenomas. The Journal of Clinical Endocrinology and Metabolism. 2000;**85**:1789-1793. DOI: 10.1210/jc.85.5.1789

[95] Capatina C, Inder W, Karavitaki N, Wass JA. Management of endocrine disease: Pituitary tumour apoplexy. European Journal of Endocrinology. 2015;**172**:R179-R190. DOI: 10.1530/EJE-14-0794

[96] Sweeney AT, Blake MA, Adelman LS, et al. Pituitary apoplexy precipitating diabetes insipidus. Endocrine Practice. 2004;**10**:135-138. DOI: 10.4158/EP.10.2.135

[97] Ebner FH, Hauser TK, Honegger J. SIADH following pituitary adenoma apoplexy. Neurological Sciences. 2010;**31**:217-218. DOI: 10.1007/s10072-009-0210-z

[98] Krull I, Christ E, Kamm CP, Ganter C, Sahli R. Hyponatremia associated coma due to pituitary apoplexy in early pregnancy: A case report. Gynecological Endocrinology. 2010;**26**:197-200. DOI: 10.3109/09513590903184118

[99] Agrawal D, Mahapatra AK. Pituitary apoplexy and inappropriate ADH secretion. Journal of Clinical Neuroscience. 2003;**10**(2):260-261. DOI: 10.1016/S0967-5868(03)00002-X

[100] Iglesias P, Diez JJ. Thyroid dysfunction and kidney disease. European Journal of Endocrinology. 2009;**160**:503-515. DOI: 10.1530/EJE-08-0837

[101] Bonneville JF, Bonneville F. Pituitary apoplexy. In: Catin F, Nagi S, editors. MRI of the Pituitary Gland. Vol. 2014. Switzerland: Springer; 2016. pp. 89-95. DOI: 10.1007/978-3-319-29043-0_13

[102] Freeman WD. Pituitary apoplexy. Neurocritical Care. 2005;**3**:174-176. DOI: 10.1385/NCC:3:2:174

[103] Semple PL, Jane JA, Lopes MBS, Laws ER. Pituitary apoplexy: Correlation between magnetic resonance imaging and histopathological results. Journal of Neurosurgery. 2008;**108**:909-915. DOI: 10.3171/JNS/2008/108/5/0909

[104] Agrawal B, Dziurzynski K, Shariar Salamat M, Baskaya M. The temporal association of sphenoid sinus mucosal thickening on MR imaging with pituitary apoplexy. Turkish Neurosurgery. 2012;**22**(6):785-790. DOI: 10.5137/1019-5149.JTN.4273-11.1

[105] Waqar M, McCreary R, Kearney T, Karabatsou K, Gnanalingham KK. Sphenoid sinus mucosal thickening in the acute phase of pituitary apoplexy. Pituitary. 2017;**20**(4):441-449. DOI: 10.1007/s11102-017-0804-z

[106] Rogg JM, Tung GA, Anderson G, Cortez S. Pituitary apoplexy: Early detection with diffusion-weighted MR imaging. AJNR. American Journal of Neuroradiology. 2002;**23**:1240-1245. http://www.ajnr.org/content/ajnr/23/7/1240

[107] Bonneville F, Cattin F, Marsot-Dupuch K, Dormont D, Bonneville JF, Chiras J. T1 signal hyperintensity in the sellar region: Spectrum of findings. Radiographics. 2006;**26**:93-113. DOI: 10.1148/rg.261055045

[108] Chanson P, Briet C, Salenave S. Médecine clinique endocrinologie et diabète. L'apoplexie hypophysaire. 2015;**78**. https://www.mced.fr/archives/mced/78/lapoplexiehypophysaire.html

[109] Baldeweg SE, Vanderpump M, Drake W, et al. Emergency management of pituitary apoplexy in adult patients. Endocrine Connections. 2016;**5**(5):12-15. DOI: 10.1530/EC-16-0057

[110] Abdulbaki A, Kanaan I. The impact of surgical timing on visual outcome in pituitary apoplexy: Literature review and case illustration. Surgical Neurology International. 2017;**8**:16. DOI: 10.4103/2152-7806.199557

[111] Tu M, Lu Q, Zhu P, Zheng W. Surgical versus non-surgical treatment for pituitary apoplexy: A systematic review and meta-analysis. Journal of the Neurological Sciences. 2016;**370**:258-262. DOI: 10.1016/j.jns.2016.09.047

[112] Briet C, Salenave S, Chanson P. Pituitary apoplexy. Endocrinology and Metabolism Clinics of North America. 2015;**44**:199-209. DOI: 10.1210/er.2015-1042

[113] Maccagnan P, Macedo CL, Kayath MJ, Nogueira RG, Abucham J. Conservative management of pituitary apoplexy: A prospective study. The Journal of Clinical Endocrinology and Metabolism. 1995;**80**:2190-2197. DOI: 10.1210/jcem.80.7.7608278

[114] Pelkonen R, Kuusisto A, Salmi J, et al. Pituitary function after pituitary apoplexy. The American Journal of Medicine. 1978;**65**:773-778. DOI: 10.1016/0002-9343(78)90795-7

[115] Chanson P, Salenave S. Conservative management of pituitary apoplexy. In: Turgut M, Mahapatra AK, Powell M, Muthukumar N, editors. Pituitary Apoplexy. Berlin, Heidelberg, Germany: Springer-Verlag; 2014. pp. 151-156

[116] Turgut M, Ozsunar Y, Basak S, Guney E, Kir E, Meteoglu I. Pituitary apoplexy: An overview of 186 cases published during the last century. Acta Neurochirurgica. 2010; **152**:749-761. DOI: 10.1007/s00701-009-0595

[117] Muthukumar N, Rossette D, Soundaram M, Senthilbabu S, Badrinarayanan T. Blindness following pituitary apoplexy: Timing of surgery and neuro-ophthalmic outcome. Journal of Clinical Neuroscience. 2008;**15**:873-879. DOI: 10.1016/j.jocn.2007.08.010

[118] Bujawansa S, Thondam SK, Steele C, et al. Presentation, management and outcomes in acute pituitary apoplexy: A large single-centre experience from the United Kingdom. Clinical Endocrinology. 2014;**80**:419-424. DOI: 10.1111/cen.12307

[119] Boellis A, di Napoli A, Romano A, Bozzao A. Pituitary apoplexy: An update on clinical and imaging features. Insights Imaging. 2014;**5**:753-762. DOI: 10.1007/s13244-014-0362-0

[120] Bi WL, Dunn IF, Laws ER. Pituitary apoplexy. Endocrine. 2015;**48**:69-75. DOI: 10.1007/s12020-014-0359

Section 4

Neuroophthalmology in Pituitary Disease

Chapter 6

Neuro-Ophthalmology Findings in Pituitary Disease (Review of Literature)

Arwa Azmeh

Additional information is available at the end of the chapter

http://dx.doi.org/10.5772/intechopen.77065

Abstract

Visual symptoms often accompany pituitary diseases. Pituitary tumors may compress surrounding structures such as optic chiasm leading to visual field defects including bitemporal hemianopia and visual disturbance. They also may compress cranial nerves III, IV, and VI, leading to ocular motility abnormalities. Pituitary adenomas are the most common cause of chiasmal compression. Patients with nonsecreting tumors present initially with vision loss, and these tumors can reach large size without causing other symptoms; however, hormonally active tumors are detected before vision loss because of systemic symptoms. Acute hemorrhage or infarction of the pituitary tumor known as pituitary apoplexy causes diplopia, loss of vision, and visual field. Thus, the ophthalmologist's role is crucial in diagnosis and treatment of pituitary tumors. As visual loss may be the first sign of recurrence after treatment, it is essential to repeat visual field and visual acuity testing every 6–12 months.

Keywords: pituitary tumors, pituitary adenoma, pituitary apoplexy, chiasmal compression, bitemporal hemianopia, ocular motility abnormalities, craniopharyngioma, suprasellar meningioma, parasellar meningioma

1. Introduction

Pituitary diseases are the most common causes of extrinsic compressive chiasmal syndromes leading to visual disturbances. Chiasmal syndromes most commonly occur secondary to pituitary adenomas, craniopharyngiomas, meningiomas, and pituitary apoplexy.

Visual field defects may be one of the first signs of nonfunctional pituitary tumors growing in the vertical direction [1]. Visual disturbances are much less frequent in functional adenomas, where systemic hormonal aberrations such as Cushing's syndrome, galactorrhea, and acromegaly usually predate the compressive signs [2].

However, pituitary tumors may grow in the horizontal direction to invade the cavernous sinus. This will cause dysfunction of cranial nerves III, IV, V, and VI, with less visual damage [1].

2. Anatomy

2.1. Optic nerve

The optic nerve extends from the retina to the optic chiasm; it is approximately 5 cm long and is divided into four portions: intraocular or optic disk (1 mm), intraorbital (25 mm), intracanalicular within the optic canal (9 mm), and intracranial which terminates in the optic chiasm (12–16 mm) [3].

2.2. Optic chiasm

The optic chiasm measures approximately 12 mm wide, 8 mm long in the anteroposterior direction, and 4 mm thick. It is inclined at almost 45°, located just anterior to the hypothalamus and anterior to the third ventricle, and situated about 10 mm above the pituitary gland, which rests in the sella turcica of the sphenoid bone. The chiasm and sella are separated by a space called the suprasellar or inferior chiasmatic cistern [4].

As a result of variations in the length of the optic nerves, the exact location of the chiasm with respect to the sella is variable [4]. Most of the time, (80%) it is central and lies directly over the sella (expanding pituitary tumors involves chiasma first). In approximately 10% of individuals, it is prefixed as it lies more anteriorly over tuberculum sellae (pituitary tumors involves optic tract first), and in approximately 10%, it is posterior (postfixed) lying more posterior over dorsum sellae (pituitary tumors damage the optic nerve) [5–8].

The pituitary infundibulum, which arises from the hypothalamus (ventral diencephalon) behind the chiasm, extends downward to the posterior lobe of the pituitary (neurohypophysis). The anterior lobe of the pituitary (adenohypophysis) forms embryologically from Rathke's pouch, an embryological structure connected to the pharynx. The chiasm is flanked laterally by the supraclinoid segments of the carotid arteries and inferolaterally by the cavernous sinuses [8, 9].

At the optic chiasm, retinal ganglion cell axons from the temporal retina remain ipsilateral, and those from the nasal retina cross the chiasm and course toward the contralateral brain [10]. However, there are intricacies in the chiasmal crossing [11]. In the process of decussating, fibers from the inferior nasal quadrant loop forward into the opposite optic nerve for a short distance before turning back again, forming Wilbrand's knee. In addition, some of the upper nasal fibers loop back briefly into the ipsilateral optic tract before decussation. In the chiasm, the fibers from the upper retinal quadrants lie superior, and those from the lower quadrants inferior. Inferior nasal fibers decussate anteriorly and inferiorly in the chiasm, while superior nasal fibers cross posteriorly and superiorly. This accounts for the difference in the pattern of evolution of the field defect in infrachiasmatic versus suprachiasmatic lesions. Macular fibers more or less decussate as a group, forming a miniature chiasm within the chiasm, primarily in the posterior superior portion [11].

2.3. Visual field testing

The primary role of the clinician in the diagnosis of chiasmal disorders is to assess visual function accurately, interpret the results correctly, and, thus, localize the anatomical region that is affected. Visual field tests may provide a strong indication of direct chiasmal involvement, and failure to perform and properly interpret visual field tests is a common cause for delay in the diagnosis of chiasmal disorders [12].

Chiasmal injury is classically associated with bitemporal visual field defects due to damage to crossing fibers that carry temporal visual field information from the nasal retinas. Retinal ganglion cell axons from either side (right or left) of the macula travel together through the optic nerve but separate at the optic chiasm. This divergence creates the hemianopic midline and is the reason that all chiasmal and retrochiasmal visual field defects respect the vertical meridian [13].

Bitemporal defects that respect the vertical meridian indicate damage to the visual pathways at the optic chiasm [14]. It is important to establish that the vertical midline forms the border of the field depression and accordingly to rule out nonchiasmal temporal field loss that does not respect the vertical midline [12].

Bitemporal hemianopias may be complete (with no vision temporal to fixation in either eye), but when compression is early or mild, the hemianopia may be denser superiorly (when the chiasm is compressed from below) or inferiorly (when the chiasm is compressed from above) [13].

Because crossing macular fibers travel posteriorly, a lesion of the posterior chiasm may result in a central bitemporal hemianopia, sparing the more peripheral temporal fields [13].

Rarely, an anterior lesion at the junction of the optic nerve and the optic chiasm can injure crossing fibers from the opposite inferior retina (which loop forward into the optic nerve, forming Wilbrand's knee, before projecting posteriorly to the optic tract). As a result, the optic nerve visual field defected in one eye may be accompanied by a superior temporal scotoma in the other eye: the junctional scotoma [13].

Lesions causing compression of the optic tract produce dissimilar incongruous homonymous defects in the hemifields contralateral to the affected optic tract [15].

3. Ophthalmologist's role in pituitary tumors

Pituitary tumors are common benign tumors that represent about 12% of intracranial tumors [12].

Studies of several old series of pituitary tumors led to the old classical ophthalmology teaching that visual field abnormalities were an important early diagnostic sign of pituitary tumor [16].

Henderson [17] reviewed Cushing's series of 338 pituitary tumors in 1939. He found that chromophobe adenoma was almost never diagnosed before it had grown large enough to compress the anterior visual pathways causing field defects. Furthermore, he felt that no operation should be undertaken unless vision was at risk. In 1955, Chamlin et al. [18] reviewed 156 cases of pituitary tumors and found that 86% of these cases had field defects. Hollenhorst et al. [19] analyzed 1000 cases of pituitary tumors, which were diagnosed between 1940 and 1962, and found visual field defects in 70% of patients. Klauber et al. [20] reviewed 51 patients with pituitary tumors seen between 1967 and 1974 and reported a 69% incidence of field defects. Wray [21] examined 100 pituitary tumor patients between 1974 and 1976 and demonstrated field defects in 31%. Anderson et al. [16] reported, in their study of 200 patients with pituitary tumors seen between 1976 and 1981, 9% incidence of field defects.

In comparing the above six studies done before 1981 and including all pituitary tumors regardless of their origin, size, and presenting symptoms, it was obvious that the incidence of ophthalmologic findings was decreasing in patients with pituitary tumors. This can be explained by the following several developments which enabled earlier diagnosis and treatment before visual disturbance had occurred [16]:

1. Availability of prolactin assays: Prior to prolactin era, though the clinical syndromes of amenorrhea/galactorrhea in women had been described in pituitary tumors, their cause was not understood, as these tumors could be identified on plain skull x-rays, only in minority of patients when they were large enough to be seen. It is not surprising then that many of these patients received no specific therapy until they developed visual field defects.

2. Progress in radiologic imaging techniques: Prior to 1980, access to high-resolution CT scanning was limited, so this examination was carried out only in patients with large visual field defects. Since 1980 development of CT scanning techniques made it possible to visualize lesions smaller than 3 to 4 mm in diameter.

3. Development of surgical techniques: Before the development of selective transsphenoidal adenectomy techniques in which only the adenoma is removed and the rest of the pituitary is left intact, surgical removal of an adenoma was accomplished transfrontally by total hypophysectomy, with the resultant higher morbidity and mortality. Since the iatrogenic hypopituitarism was a major medical problem, surgical removal of pituitary adenomas was often not recommended until visual manifestations developed.

As a result of these developments, the ophthalmologist's role in the diagnosis of pituitary tumors appeared to be changing from the classical teaching [16]. Patients became less likely to present primarily because of visual complaints but more likely to be referred to the ophthalmologist by an endocrinologist, gynecologist, or neurosurgeon during the course of a workup of a suspected pituitary tumor. However, for the small group of nonsecreting tumors, the ophthalmologist still has a primary role in that these patients will often present first with field defects.

Later on Poon et al. [22] performed a prospective study on 29 patients with visual deficits who presented to the neurosurgical unit for removal of pituitary macroadenomas between

1992 and 1994. All patients had visual field defects. It is noteworthy that out of the 29 patients, only 11 (37.9%) were referred by an ophthalmologist, which means that visual disturbance and visual field defects were the first presenting symptoms in only 37.9% of patients with macroadenomas. Other patients were referred by general practitioners, neurologists, endocrinologists, gynecologists, general physicians, and optometrists in 34.5, 10.3, 6.8, 3.4, 3.4, and 3.4%, respectively.

Ren-Wen Ho et al. [1] reviewed retrospectively the records of 78 patients with pituitary adenomas who were referred for transsphenoidal adenectomy between 2009 and 2011. Among these patients, 24 had small macroadenomas (>1 cm to ≤2 cm), 37 had large macroadenoma (>2 cm to ≤4 cm), and 17 had giant adenomas (>4 cm). Abnormal visual fields were found in 65.4% of all patients. Patients with large macroadenomas and giant adenomas had a higher rate of abnormal visual field in comparison with patients with small macroadenomas (81.1, 94.1, and 20.8%, respectively).

The increase in incidence of visual field defects in patients with pituitary tumors in reports published after the 1980s (varies from 65.4–100%) [1, 22] may be explained by the fact that recent studies were more specific and included in general only patients with macroadenomas, who were referred to neurologists for transsphenoidal adenectomy (these patients are more susceptible to have visual field defects), while reports before 1980s were more general and included all pituitary tumors regardless of their size, presenting symptoms, and indication for surgery.

Another way in which patients with pituitary tumors may present to the ophthalmologist is investigation of ocular causes of headache. Besides searching for primary ocular causes of headache, the ophthalmologist should be aware of performing careful visual fields in all headache patients. In addition to performing careful visual field examinations on routine headache patients, the ophthalmologist must be willing to question these patients about reproductive and sexual dysfunction and to refer these patients for appropriate neuroendocrine and neuroradiologic investigation [16].

4. Pituitary adenomas

Pituitary adenomas make up 12–15% of symptomatic intracranial neoplasms [12]. They are the most common causes of chiasmal compression and may occur at any adult age; they are rare in childhood [15].

Typically, nonfunctioning adenomas present as macroadenomas that cause neurological symptoms due to intracranial mass effects, since hormonal inactivity leads to a delay in diagnosis compared with functioning pituitary adenomas [23]. If pituitary adenomas are not treated, vision will continue to deteriorate and blindness might result [24].

A relationship exists between severity of visual impairment and tumor size [25]. Pituitary adenomas are usually classified into microadenomas, macroadenomas, and giant adenomas according to their size [26–29]. The larger the pituitary adenoma is, the higher is the risk of optic chiasm or optic nerve compression [16, 19, 30]. In general, the size of macroadenomas range from 1 to 4 cm. Smaller macroadenomas typically will not result in any visual field defect or visual impairment, whereas the larger ones will usually cause severe visual disability. Several studies clearly illustrated that patients with larger tumors tended to have visual field abnormality and that the severity of visual field defects was closely related to tumor size [31, 32]. Investigation of the relation between the severity of the visual impairment and the different sizes of macroadenomas by Ren-Wen Ho et al. [1] indicated that pituitary adenomas less than 2 cm usually have no or only a minimal effect on the visual pathway.

The typical visual field defect, bitemporal hemianopia, is due to the anatomical compression of the optic chiasm, which contains the crossing nasal fibers of each optic nerve. Nevertheless, the visual field defect actually depends on the relation between the optic chiasm and the tumor itself. If the tumor is anterior to the optic chiasm, or if the patient has an anatomical postfixed chiasm, conditions such as central scotoma, arcuate scotoma, and monocular visual constriction can be noted. If the tumor compresses the optic tracts, or the patient has a prefixed chiasm, a homonymous hemianopia might be seen [31, 33, 34].

Ren-Wen Ho et al. [1] found that large macroadenomas and giant adenomas leading to visual impairment are mostly nonfunctioning adenomas (97.8%). This result is consistent with other reports [16, 35] and can be explained by the absence of endocrine symptoms, which often result in a delay of the diagnosis since there are no early visual symptoms [16]. This explanation is consistent with what Monteiro et al. [32] have mentioned previously that nonfunctioning and prolactin-secreting adenomas are the most likely pituitary tumors associated with visual impairment.

In general, larger volume tumors will usually result in a higher risk of compression at the optic chiasm; however, this relationship is not found when tumor extension mainly occurs at the infrasellar or parasellar region instead of the suprasellar region. It was found that if the adenoma grows in the vertical direction, it will usually result in more severe visual impairment. If the adenoma grows in the horizontal direction, it will usually cause less vision damage. Horizontal growth of the adenoma may invade the cavernous sinus [1].

Furthermore, some studies have already discussed the relationship between the optic chiasm position and visual loss. Ikeda and Yoshimoto [36] found that visual impairment occurred when the displacement of the optic chiasm was more than 8 mm above the reference line on the sagittal image and more than 13 mm above on the coronal image on brain MRI. Monteiro et al. [32] have also shown that tumor exceeding 10 mm above the sagittal standard line and 12 mm above the coronal standard line had a significant effect on visual loss. Ren-Wen Ho et al. [1] found that significant visual impairment occurred when the optic chiasm was moved by the tumor more than 11.2 mm above the reference line on the sagittal view and more than 15.3 mm on the coronal image.

With regard to visual improvement after surgery for pituitary adenoma, Ren-Wen Ho et al. [1] reported visual improvement in 88.7% with complete recovery of vision in 27.67% of patients. They found that patients with large macroadenomas or giant adenomas experienced greater visual improvement after surgical resection compared with patients who had micro- or small macroadenomas, but patients with smaller pituitary adenomas still had a better visual outcome. Other series have reported that visual improvement depends on the surgical approach, ranging from 74.7 to 93.4% [24, 37, 38]. Gnanalingham et al. [35] believed that better preoperative visual acuity and a smaller degree of impairment in preoperative visual field would have a better effect on the visual outcome.

There have been contradictory results regarding predictive factors for recovery of vision. Müslüman et al. [24] found that tumor size was not significantly associated with the postoperative visual impairment score, but preoperative visual deficit and the time interval between the initial visual symptom and surgery were the factors significantly associated with the postoperative visual impairment score. A shorter duration of symptoms, younger age, and a better preoperative best-corrected visual acuity (BCVA) have been reported to be associated with better postoperative recovery of visual field by some investigators [35].

Undoubtedly, vision can rapidly improve within minutes or days after tumor resection [39]. Among all surgical resection procedures, transsphenoidal adenectomy is likely most effective for providing rapid relief of visual symptoms in patients with a pituitary adenoma [40, 41]. Thus, early surgical resection of the tumor should be considered for patients with a large or giant macroadenoma causing visual loss, in order to preserve their vision.

5. Pituitary apoplexy

Pituitary apoplexy is the sudden enlargement of a pituitary gland, as a result from hemorrhage or infarction (most commonly hemorrhagic infarction) of a pituitary adenoma [42]. Pituitary apoplexy is typically associated with acute headache, visual field or vision loss, ophthalmoplegia, facial pain, or facial numbness.

Sudden expansion of the tumor into the adjacent cavernous sinuses can cause dysfunction of cranial nerves III, IV, V, and VI, with cranial nerve III as the most commonly affected one. Superior extension causes visual field loss; it also may cause central visual loss up to no light perception vision. Extravasation of blood into the subarachnoid space causes numerous symptoms, including a decreased level of consciousness and vasospasm with secondary stroke. The acute endocrine abnormalities may lead to numerous complications, including adrenal crisis. Therefore, recognition of pituitary apoplexy is crucial, as treatment is initiated emergently. Treatment includes immediate administration of corticosteroids, surgical decompression of the sella, and appropriate supportive measures. Some authorities recommend conservative management when neuro-ophthalmic signs are absent or mild [15].

The normal pituitary gland also may undergo hemorrhagic or nonhemorrhagic infarction, but such episodes generally do not cause visual loss and may go unrecognized until hypopituitarism develops. Predisposing factors include pregnancy, estrogen therapy, obstetrical hemorrhage (Sheehan's syndrome), diabetes mellitus, bleeding disorders, long-term anticoagulation, blood dyscrasias, radiation therapy, trauma, angiography, atheromatous emboli, cardiac surgery, coughing, positive pressure ventilation, and vasoactive agents [12].

As presentation of acute pituitary apoplexy is variable and its course is unpredictable, it should be considered in any patient with abrupt neuro-ophthalmological deterioration associated with headache. Although early investigators suggested that pituitary apoplexy occurs primarily in patients with large macroadenomas, it is now evident that tumors of almost any size may undergo hemorrhagic necrosis [43, 44].

6. Lymphocytic adenohypophysitis

Lymphocytic adenohypophysitis is an immune-mediated diffuse lymphocytic infiltration of the pituitary gland; it has been reported to cause chiasmal compression from suprasellar extension [45]. This uncommon condition was reported in women only, and over one-half of the cases was found to occur during the perinatal period.

7. Craniopharyngioma

Craniopharyngiomas comprise 3% of all intracranial tumors, 13% of intracranial neoplasms in childhood, and 30% of all new growths in the hypophyseal area [46]. Since ocular signs are frequently the presenting features of these tumors, it is clear that their recognition by ophthalmologist is of great importance for establishing early diagnosis and treatment and more favorable prognosis.

Craniopharyngioma is a benign tumor, of ectodermal origin, arising from squamous cell remnants of Rathke's pouch. These cell remnants occur mainly on the infundibulum, between the undersurface of the brain and the upper surface of the pituitary gland [46]. The tumor may be entirely suprasellar or partially intrasellar, resulting in avascular solid tissue mass in which calcification may occur, as well as cysts filled with cellular debris and cholesterol crystals [46]. About 90% of tumors contain cysts, some of which may be very large [47]. These tumors may produce variable symptoms and signs depending on their size, direction of growth, and degree of compression of the optic pathways, pituitary area, hypothalamus, and third ventricle.

One of the striking features in craniopharyngioma is the variation in visual acuity and visual field loss, observed with disease progression [46]. Thus, information should be gathered from repeated field testing rather than from any single measurement [46]. These fluctuations can occur in both solid tumors (perhaps due to local edema) and in cystic variety (from intermittent emptying of the cyst into the ventricles) [48].

Kennedy and Smith [46] found in their study of 45 patients with craniopharyngioma that the majority of adults presented with visual failure and optic atrophy. Bitemporal hemianopia was fairly frequent (found in 27% of patients at the time of diagnosis) but was asymmetrical and unpredictable in its evolution. Homonymous hemianopia was relatively common (found as presenting feature in 11% of patients). Full fields were found initially in 20% of patients, a high incidence compared with pituitary adenomas or suprasellar meningiomas. Furthermore, Kennedy and Smith [46] detected pleomorphism (a distinct change from one type of field defect to another, with progress of the disease), which is a characteristic feature of the tumor (as indeed are fluctuations in the clinical state and visual acuity), in 22% of their patients.

In children, there are two main presenting syndromes [48]: (1) symptoms and signs of raised intracranial pressure, resulting from obstruction of the third ventricle by the tumor, and (2) visual failure from compression of the visual pathways. Kennedy and Smith [46] pointed out that, in those patients who have raised intracranial pressure, optic atrophy may be found rather than papilledema.

In addition, strabismus is a common finding in craniopharyngioma patients, and it can be classified into three categories [46, 49]:

1. Cases of concomitant esotropia or exotropia following marked loss of central vision in one or both eyes:

Kennedy and Smith [46] reported this type of squint as an early feature of craniopharyngioma in 30% of children included in their study. As the presence of optic atrophy or sluggish pupil may be missed in a young child, the poor vision in the squinting eye may be wrongly attributed to strabismic amblyopia until it is realized that the visual acuity is deteriorating despite treatment.

2. Cases of paralytic strabismus:

The incidence of paralytic strabismus was variable between different case series of craniopharyngioma. Love and Marshall [49] found in year 1950 third nerve palsy in 10% of their cases, while Hoff and Patterson reported in 1972 the incidence of cranial nerve palsies in 25% of children and 33% of adults [46]. Wybar found in 1971 two cases of third nerve palsy and one case of sixth nerve palsy, in 72 cases [46]. Kennedy and Smith [46] had only one patient in their series with transient sixth nerve paresis and were surprised not to have more cases of ophthalmoplegia, in spite of the massive size of the cystic tumor present in many of their craniopharyngioma patients.

3. Cases of non-paretic diplopia:

It is characterized by episodes of diplopia in the absence of demonstrable ocular palsy or defect of ocular movement [46], which was attributed to disturbance of binocular vision, secondary to bitemporal hemianopia and reduction of the area of visual field overlap common to the two eyes.

Endocrine disorders are also common in craniopharyngioma especially in adults, and mental deterioration is a frequent presenting feature in patients over 30 years of age [46]. Straight x-rays of the skull are practically diagnostic of craniopharyngioma in children, but in adults a normal x-ray does not exclude the diagnosis.

8. Sellar and suprasellar meningiomas

Meningiomas in the region of the sella turcica are rare, representing about 1% of all sellar masses [50]. They typically originate and involve the suprasellar region but in unusual cases arise from within the sella. Sellar/suprasellar meningiomas can mimic both clinically and radiologically, any of the other nonhormone-secreting sellar region masses, in particular the nonfunctioning pituitary adenomas. They can cause loss of visual acuity, visual field disturbances, hypopituitarism, hyperprolactinemia, or a combination of the above [51].

Kwancharoen et al. [52] analyzed a retrospective series of subset of 44 patients with sellar/suprasellar meningiomas and adequate MRI imaging study, who underwent surgery at the Johns Hopkins Hospital during a 12-year period (between 2000 and 2012). They were mostly diagnosed in the sixth decade (age ranges between 30 and 78 years). The female/male ratio was 6:1, quite higher than the reported one in the previous series and higher than the ratio found in the entire meningioma cohort (2.7:1) [53–55]. The most common presenting symptoms were visual disturbance (85.96%), although some series report them in an even higher proportion (82.4–100%) [53, 54], and this was followed by headaches (49.12%), diplopia (12.28%), and ptosis (7.02%). A small proportion of patients had symptoms of endocrine dysfunction. Among these, hyperprolactinemia was the most common one, highlighting the fact that prolactin can be above the threshold in nonprolactin-secreting sellar masses. An additional meningioma was found in two cases (3.5%), one in the region of the falx cerebri and one in the middle cranial fossa [52].

MRI is the investigation of choice in these cases because it can often show the dural origin of the tumor [52]. In agreement with the previous series [56, 57], most of the tumors (81.25%) reported by Kwancharoen et al. [52] were iso-intense in T1. On T2-weighted imaging, the tumors were hyperintense in 35%, iso-intense in 30%, and hypointense in 25% of the cases [52].

Due to the high vascularity, gadolinium enhancement of meningiomas is usually marked, homogeneous, and rapid [58, 59]. This enhancement pattern may be helpful in distinguishing them from adenomas. However, in Kwancharoen et al.'s sellar/suprasellar series [52] in almost 11% of cases, the mass was thought to be a pituitary adenoma. This fact points out the significant challenges of establishing the diagnosis through radiology alone and necessitates further work to establish more accurate clinical and radiologic means of distinguishing between meningiomas and macroadenomas in the region of the sella turcica.

Because of the fibrous content in histology and expression of angiogenesis factors, meningiomas are usually adhesive, firm, and high vascular and may have major intraoperative bleeding and worse surgical outcome when compared to pituitary adenomas [60].

Previous series report worsening of vision in approximately 20–30% after surgery for sellar and parasellar meningiomas [53, 61–63]. Kwancharoen et al. [52] found deterioration of vision in 10.5% of cases after surgery (79.6% had improvement of one or more symptoms, improvement of vision occurred in 79.6%, and improvement of headache in 7.14%). It was proposed that surgical techniques might affect this outcome, as optic nerve manipulation and devascularization of perforating arteries supplying the optic apparatus are important factors for visual outcome [63, 64]. As Kwancharoen et al. [52] reported outcomes of more recent surgeries, the lower prevalence of vision deterioration when compared with previous reports might reflect the historical improvement in surgical techniques.

9. Parasellar meningiomas

Parasellar meningiomas occur most often in middle-aged women; arise most frequently from the tuberculum sella, planum sphenoidale, or anterior clinoid; and often produce asymmetric bitemporal vision loss. Parasellar meningiomas may also enlarge and produce chiasmal compression during pregnancy [15].

Parasellar involvement manifests with abnormalities of ocular motility, pupillary function, or facial sensation from injury to cranial nerves III, IV, V1, V2, or VI or the ocular sympathetic nerves in the parasellar region [12]. Injury to these structures within the cavernous sinus may be associated with complaints of diplopia, ptosis, unequal pupil size, accommodative difficulty, facial pain or numbness, or eye pain. Signs include ocular motor nerve palsies, decreased sensation in the areas innervated by the first and second divisions of the trigeminal nerve, or Horner's syndrome [12]. Multiple cranial nerve involvement is more suggestive of invasive malignant tumors [12].

Therapy of parasellar tumors is complex and depends on the age of the patient; the nature, location, and extent of the tumor; its hormonal activity; and the severity of symptoms [15].

The ophthalmologist's role in the management of parasellar tumors is crucial, in that the first sign of recurrence may be vision loss [15]. Baseline visual field and visual acuity testing should be performed 2–3 months after treatment and at intervals of 6–12 months thereafter, depending on the course. Visual acuity and visual fields should be rechecked more often (immediately if necessary) if the patient notes any ongoing change. Periodic neuroimaging is essential [15].

Delayed vision loss after therapy for parasellar lesions should prompt the following considerations [15]:

- Tumor recurrence.
- Delayed radio necrosis of the chiasm or optic nerves.
- Chiasmal distortion due to adhesions or secondary empty sella syndrome, with traction on the chiasm.
- Chiasmal compression from expansion of intraoperative over packing of the sella with fat.

Neuroimaging effectively helps differentiate among these entities and guides further management decisions [15].

10. Conclusion

Due to developments in laboratory assays, radiological imaging, and surgical techniques, patients with pituitary tumors became less likely to present primarily to the ophthalmologist because of visual complaints. These patients are more likely referred to ophthalmologists by the endocrinologist, gynecologist, or neurosurgeon at earlier stages of pituitary disease during the course of workup. However, the ophthalmologist still has a primary role in patients with nonsecreting tumors, where patients will present first with visual and field defects. Patients with pituitary apoplexy usually present with acute headache, visual field or vision loss, ophthalmoplegia, facial pain, or facial numbness. In craniopharyngioma, strabismus is a common finding. It can be concomitant or paralytic. In addition, the patient may complain of non-paretic diplopia. The most common presenting sign in sellar/suprasellar meningiomas is visual disturbance, followed by headaches, diplopia, and ptosis. Parasellar meningiomas manifest with ocular motility abnormalities, abnormal pupillary reaction, as well as abnormal facial sensation; these complaints result from injury to cranial nerves III, IV, V1, V2, or VI and ocular sympathetic nerves in the parasellar region.

Author details

Arwa Azmeh

Address all correspondence to: arwaretina@gmail.com

Almouassat University Hospital, Damascus University, Damascus, Syria

References

[1] Ho R-W, Huang H-M, Ho J-T. The influence of pituitary adenoma size on vision and visual outcomes after trans-sphenoidal adenectomy: A report of 78 cases. Journal of Korean Neurosurgical Association. 2015;**57**(1):23-31. DOI: 10.3340/jkns.2015.57.1.23. PMCID: PMC4323501

[2] Wikipedia, the Free Encyclopedia [Internet]. 2018. Available from https://en.wikipedia.org/wiki/Pituitary_adenoma [Accessed: 2018-03-19]

[3] Myron Y, Jay D, editors. Ophthalmology. 4th ed. Philadelphia: Saunders; 2014. pp. 866-868

[4] American Academy of Ophthalmology. Basic and clinical science course section 5. Neuro-Ophthalmology; **2013-2014**:28-29

[5] Campero A, Martins C, Yasuda A, Rhoton AL Jr. Microsurgical anatomy of the diaphragma sellae and its role in directing the pattern of growth of pituitary adenomas. Journal of Neurosurgery. 2008;**62**(3):717-723

[6] Glaser JS, editor. Neuro-Ophthalmology: Symposium of the University of Miami and the Bascom Palmer Eye Institute. Vol. 9. St Louis: CV Mosby; 1977. pp. 75-105

[7] Bergland RM, Ray BS, Torack RM. Anatomical variations in the pituitary gland and adjacent structures in 225 autopsy cases. Journal of Neurosurgery. 1968;**28**(2):93-99

[8] Chin BM, Orlandi RR, Wiggins RH 3rd. Evaluation of the sellar and parasellar regions. Magnetic Resonance Imaging Clinics of North America. 2012;**20**(3):515-543

[9] Warwick R, editor. Eugene Wolff's Anatomy of the Eye and Orbit. 7th ed. Philadelphia: WB Saunders; 1976. pp. 406-417

[10] Levin L, Nilsson S, Ver Hoeve J, Wu S, editors. Adler's Physiology of the Eye. 11th ed. Philadelphia: Saunders; 2011. p. 552

[11] Neupsy Key Fastest Neupsy Insight Engine [Internet]. 2016. Available from: https://neupsykey.com/the-optic-nerve-4/# [Accessed: 2016-12-16]

[12] Myron Y, Jay D, editors. Ophthalmology. 4th ed. Philadelphia: Saunders; 2014. pp. 900-908

[13] Neupsy Key Fastest Neupsy Insight Engine [Internet]. 2016. Available from: https://neupsykey.com/eye-signs-in-neurologic-diagnosis [Accessed: 2016-09-08]

[14] Levin L, Nilsson S, Ver Hoeve J, Wu S editors. Adler's Physiology of the Eye. 11th ed. Philadelphia: Saunders; 2011. p 664

[15] American Academy of Ophthalmology. Basic and clinical science course section 5. Neuro-Ophthalmology; **2013-2014**:146-153

[16] Anderson D, Faber P, Marcovitz S, Hardy J, Lorenzetii D. Pituitary tumors and the ophthalmologist. Ophthalmology. 1983;**90**(11):1265-1270

[17] Henderson WR. The pituitary adenomata, a follow-up study of the surgical results in 338 cases. The British Journal of Surgery. 1939;**26**:811-921

[18] Chamlin M, Davidoff LM, Feiring EH. Ophthalmological changes produced by pituitary tumors. American Journal of Ophthalmology. 1955;**40**:353-368

[19] Hollenhorst RW, Younge BR. Ocular manifestations produced by adenomas of the pituitary gland: Analysis of 1000 cases. In: Kohler PO, Ross GT, editors. Diagnosis and Treatment of Pituitary Tumours. (International Congress Series no. 303). Amsterdam: Excerpta Medica; 1973. pp. 53-68

[20] Klauber A, Rasmussen P, Lindholm J. Pituitary adenoma and visual function; the prognostic value of clinical, ophthalmological and neuroradiologic findings in 51 patients subjected to operation. Acta Ophthalmologica. 1978;**56**:252-563

[21] Wray SH. Neuro-ophthalmologic manifestations of pituitary and parasellar lesions. Clinical Neurosurgery. 1976;**24**:86-117

[22] Poon A, McNeill P, Harper A, O'Day J. Patterns of visual loss associated with pituitary macroadenomas. Australian and New Zeland Jurnal of Ophthalmology. 1993;**23**(2):107-115

[23] Colao A, Di Somma C, Pivonello R, Faggiano A, Lombardi G, Savastano S. Medical therapy for clinically non-functioning pituitary adenomas. Endocrine-Related Cancer. 2008;**15**(4):905-915

[24] Müslüman AM, Cansever T, Yılmaz A, Kanat A, Oba E, ÇavuŞoğlu H, Sirinoğlu D, Aydın Y. Surgical results of large and giant pituitary adenomas with special consideration of ophthalmologic outcomes. World Neurosurgery. 2011;**76**:141-148

[25] Thomas R, Shenoy K, Seshadri MS, Muliyil J, Rao A, Paul P. Visual field defects in non-functioning pituitary adenomas. Indian Journal of Ophthalmology. 2002;**50**(2):127-130

[26] Garibi J, Pomposo I, Villar G, Gaztambide S. Giant pituitary adenomas: Clinical characteristics and surgical results. British Journal of Neurosurgery. 2002;**16**(2):133-139

[27] Goel A, Nadkarni T, Muzumdar D, Desai K, Phalke U, Sharma P. Giant pituitary tumors: A study based on surgical treatment of 118 cases. Surgical Neurology. 2004;**61**:436-445

[28] Hennessey JV, Jackson IM. Clinical features and differential diagnosis of pituitary tumours with emphasis on acromegaly. Baillière's Clinical Endocrinology and Metabolism. 1995;**9**(2):271-314

[29] Krisht AF. Giant invasive pituitary adenomas: Management plan. Contemporary Neurosurgery. 1999;**21**:1-6

[30] Ebersold MJ, Quast LM, Laws ER, Jr, Scheithauer B, Randall RV: Long-term results in transsphenoidal removal of nonfunctioning pituitary adenomas. Journal of Neurosurgery 1986;**64**(5):713-719

[31] Rivoal O, Brézin AP, Feldman-Billard S, Luton JP. Goldmann perimetry in acromegaly: A survey of 307 cases from 1951 through 1996. Ophthalmology. 2000;**107**:991-997

[32] Monteiro ML, Zambon BK, Cunha LP. Predictive factors for the development of visual loss in patients with pituitary macroadenomas and for visual recovery after optic pathway decompression. Canadian Journal of Ophthalmology. 2010;**45**:404-408

[33] Foroozan R. Chiasmal syndromes. Current Opinion in Ophthalmology. 2003;**14**(6):325-331

[34] Nishimura M, Kurimoto T, Yamagata Y, Ikemoto H, Arita N, Mimura O. Giant pituitary adenoma manifesting as homonymous hemianopia. Japanese Journal of Ophthalmology. 2007;**51**:151-153

[35] Gnanalingham KK, Bhattacharjee S, Pennington R, Ng J, Mendoza N. The time course of visual field recovery following transphenoidal surgery for pituitary adenomas: Predictive factors for a good outcome. Journal of Neurology, Neurosurgery, and Psychiatry. 2005;**76**:415-419

[36] Ikeda H, Yoshimoto T. Visual disturbances in patients with pituitary adenoma. Acta Neurologica Scandinavica. 1995;**92**(2):157-160

[37] Mortini P, Barzaghi R, Losa M, Boari N, Giovanelli M. Surgical treatment of giant pituitary adenomas: Strategies and results in a series of 95 consecutive patients. Neurosurgery. 2007;**60**(6):993-1002

[38] Zhang X, Fei Z, Zhang J, Fu L, Zhang Z, Liu W, Chen Y. Management of nonfunctioning pituitary adenomas with suprasellar extensions by transsphenoidal microsurgery. Surgical Neurology. 1999;**52**:380-385

[39] Kerrison JB, Lynn MJ, Baer CA, Newman SA, Biousse V, Newman NJ. Stages of improvement in visual fields after pituitary tumor resection. American Journal of Ophthalmology. 2000;**130**:813-820

[40] Ciric I, Ragin A, Baumgartner C, Pierce D. Complications of transsphenoidal surgery: Results of a national survey, review of the literature, and personal experience. Neurosurgery. 1997;**40**:225-236

[41] Wilson CB. Surgical management of pituitary tumors. The Journal of Clinical Endocrinology and Metabolism. 1997;**82**(8):2381-2385

[42] Wakai S, Fukushima T, Teramoto A, Sano K. Pituitary apoplexy: Its incidence and clinical significance. Journal of Neurosurgery. 1981;**55**(2):187-193

[43] Onesti ST, Wisniewski T, Post KD. Clinical versus subclinical pituitary apoplexy: Presentation, surgical management, and outcome in 21 patients. Neurosurgery. 1990;**26**(6):980-986

[44] Scheithauer BW, Gaffey TA, Lloyd RV, Sebo TJ, Kovacs KT, Horvath E, Yapicier O, Young WF Jr, Meyer FB, Kuroki T, Riehle DL, Laws ER Jr: Pathobiology of pituitary adenomas and carcinomas. Neurosurgery. 2006;**59**(2):341-353

[45] Baskin DS, Townsend JJ, Wilson CB. Lymphocytic adenohypophysitis of pregnancy simulating a pituitary adenoma: A distinct pathological entity. Journal of Neurosurgery. 1982;**56**:148-153

[46] Kennedy HB, Smith JS. Eye signs in craniopharyngioma. British Journal of Ophthalmology. 1975;**59**:689-695

[47] Jennett WB. An Introduction to Neurosurgery. 2nd ed. London: Heinemann; 1970. p. 143

[48] Russell RWR, Pennybacker JB. Craniopharyngioma in the elderly. Journal of Neurology, Neurosurgery, and Psychiatry. 1961;**24**:1-13

[49] Love JG, Marshall TM. Craniopharyngiomas (Pituitary Adamantinomas). Surgery, Gynecology & Obstetrics. 1950;**90**:591

[50] Gutenberg A, Landek-Salgado M, Tzou S, Lupi I, Geis A, Kimura H, Caturegli P. Autoimmune hypophysitis: Expanding the differential diagnosis to CTLA-4 blockade. Expert Review of Endocrinology and Metabolism. 2009;**4**(6):681-698

[51] Nozaki K, Nagata I, Yoshida K, Kikuchi H. Intrasellar meningioma: Case report and review of the literature. Surgical Neurology. 1997;**47**(5):447-452

[52] Kwancharoen R, Blitz AM, Tavares F, Caturegli P, Gallia GL, Salvatori R. Clinical Features of Sellar and Suprasellar Meningiomas. New York: Springer; 2013. DOI: 10.1007/s11102-013-0507-z

[53] Sathananthan M, Sathananthan A, Scheithauer BW, Giannini C, Meyer FB, Atkinson JL, Erickson D. Sellar meningiomas: An endocrinologic perspective. Pituitary. 2013;**16**(2): 182-188

[54] Zevgaridis D, Medele RJ, Muller A, Hischa AC, Steiger HJ. Meningiomas of the sellar region presenting with visual impairment: Impact of various prognostic factors on surgical outcome in 62 patients. Acta Neurochirurgica. 2001;**143**(5):471-476

[55] Galal A, Faisal A, Al-Werdany M, El Shehaby A, Lotfy T, Moharram H. Determinants of postoperative visual recovery in suprasellar meningiomas. Acta Neurochirurgica. 2010;**152**(1):69-77

[56] Al-Mefty O, editor. MRI of Intracranial Meningiomas. New York: Raven Press; 1991. pp. 209-223

[57] FitzPatrick M, Tartaglino LM, Hollander MD, Zimmerman RA, Flanders AE. Imaging of sellar and parasellar pathology. Radiologic Clinics of North America. 1999;**37**(1):101-121

[58] Donovan JL, Nesbit GM. Distinction of masses involving the Sella and suprasellar space: Specificity of imaging features. American Journal of Roentgenology. 1996;**167**(3):597-603

[59] Satoh H, Arita K, Kurisu K, Sumida M, Nakahara T, Eguchi K, Kuroki K. Intrasellar meningioma: Characteristic imaging findings. Neuroradiology. 1996;**38**(4):328-329

[60] Sheehan MT, Atkinson JL, Kasperbauer JL, Erickson BJ, Nippoldt TB. Preliminary comparison of the endoscopic transnasal vs the sublabial transseptal approach for clinically nonfunctioning pituitary macroadenomas. Mayo Clinic Proceedings. 1999;**74**(7):661-670

[61] Bassiouni H, Asgari S, Stolke D. Tuberculum sellae meningiomas: Functional outcome in a consecutive series treated microsurgically. Surgical Neurology. 2006;**66**(1):37-44

[62] Park CK, Jung HW, Yang SY, Seol HJ, Paek SH, Kim DG. Surgically treated tuberculum sellae and diaphragm sellae meningiomas: The importance of short-term visual outcome. Neurosurgery. 2006;**59**(2):238-243

[63] Hayhurst C, Teo C. Tuberculum sella meningioma. Otolaryngologic Clinics of North America. 2011;**44**(4):953-963

[64] Couldwell WT, Weiss MH, Rabb C, Liu JK, Apfelbaum RI, Fukushima T. Variations on the standard transsphenoidal approach to the sellar region, with emphasis on the extended approaches and parasellar approaches: Surgical experience in 105 cases. Neurosurgery. 2004;**55**(3):539-547

Section 5

Immunohistochemistry Studies

Chapter 7

Hormone Secretion in Pituitary Adenomas: Immunohistochemical Studies

Raydeh Al Khani

Additional information is available at the end of the chapter

http://dx.doi.org/10.5772/intechopen.81590

Abstract

Classification of pituitary adenomas is still changing and not completely satisfying. Various types of hormones, prehormonal substances, and transcription factors are detected in pituitary adenomas. Monohormonal secretion in pituitary adenomas is frequent, notably prolactin secretion. Secretion of more than one hormone normally originating from the same adenohypophyseal cell lineage is well known, classically GH-PRL and FSH-LH. Other combinations of hormonal secretion are reported; they are sometimes underestimated. Plurihormonal secretion in pituitary adenomas, which is secretion of hormones that are normally originating from different adenohypophyseal cell lineages, is usually underestimated and in most cases remains subclinical. An immunohistochemical study of all pituitary hormones and prehormonal substances, as demonstrating transcription factors, is not always available; it is frequently not performed. This chapter aims to show the underestimated and vague areas of pituitary adenomas and to emphasize the importance of immunohistochemical studies in the diagnosis and prediction of clinical outcomes of these adenomas.

Keywords: pituitary adenoma, monohormonal adenoma, plurihormonal adenoma, atypical adenoma, aggressive adenoma, high-risk adenoma, pituitary neuroendocrine tumor, pituitary carcinoma, immunohistochemical studies

1. Introduction

Classification of pituitary adenomas is still changing; it requires morphological and hormonal immunohistochemical assessments. These adenomas reveal various histopathological patterns and tinctorial properties which proved to be unreliable and do not always correlate with the functional or immunohistochemical findings.

The 3rd WHO classification of pituitary adenomas [1]	The 4th WHO classification of pituitary adenomas [3]
Growth hormone producing adenoma	Somatotroph adenoma
Prolactin producing adenoma	Lactotroph adenoma
Thyrotropin producing adenoma	Thyrotroph adenoma
ACTH producing adenoma	Corticotroph adenoma
Gonadotropin producing adenoma	Gonadotroph adenoma
Null cell adenoma	Null cell adenoma
Plurihormonal adenoma	Plurihormonal and double adenoma

Table 1. Comparison between the 3rd and the 4th WHO classification of pituitary adenomas.

The 3rd WHO classification of adenohypophyseal cell lineage in pituitary adenomas in 2004 was based on functional properties using histological study, immunohistochemical properties, ultrastructural features, biochemical imaging, and surgical findings [1].

The 4th WHO classification of pituitary adenomas in 2017 [2] is mostly based on the adenohypophyseal cell lineage designation according to immunohistochemical markers such as pituitary hormones and pituitary-specific transcription factors. Comparison between the 3rd and the 4th WHO classification is shown in **Table 1**.

Some transcription factors and cofactors have a known role in the differentiation of pituitary cell lineages [2–4], e.g., PIT1 (pituitary transcription factor 1 for growth hormone also known as POUF1 [3]), ER-alpha (nuclear estrogen receptor alpha), SF1 (splicing factor 1), and TPIT (transcription factor for pituitary corticotroph cell lineage).

Many adenomas secrete one hormone; though secretion of more than one hormone is well documented, the following combinations of hormones are reported [1, 3]:

- GH (growth hormone) and PRL (prolactin)
- FSH and LH
- FSH, LH, TSH, and a-SU (alpha subunit is identical for gonadotropin hormones and TSH)

Tumor cells in these cases are originating from the same cell lineage.

2. Value of immunohistochemical studies in pituitary adenomas

Immunostaining is achieving a progressively important role in pituitary adenomas. The 4th WHO classification of pituitary adenomas in 2017 [2] is mostly based on the adenohypophyseal cell lineage designation according to immunohistochemical markers for the main secreting hormones; for example, the new designation "somatotroph adenoma" defines a group of tumors that are derived from a PIT1 lineage and secrete growth hormone; this replaces the former term growth hormone-producing adenoma as previously designed in the 3rd WHO classification [1].

Immunohistochemical markers allow for differentiation between clinically relevant histological subtypes that was mainly ultrastructural features. Electron microscopy is now rarely used to classify pituitary tumors; it is not necessary for the routine investigation of pituitary tumors. However, ultrastructural evaluation may be useful in the differential diagnosis of undifferentiated tumors and in a very limited number of adenoma subtypes, such as plurihormonal PIT1-positive adenoma [2].

Transcription factors for pituitary cell lineages are as follows [3, 4]:

- Somatotroph lineage: PIT1, which is a pituitary transcription factor 1 for growth hormone also known as POUF1.
- Lactotroph differentiation: PIT1 and ER-alpha.
- Thyrotroph differentiation: PIT1 and GATA2. GATA2 is a nuclear protein regulating gene expression.
- Gonadotroph differentiation: GATA2 and SF1. SF1 is splicing factor 1, also known as zinc finger protein 162.
- Corticotroph cell lineage: TPIT.

3. Plurihormonal pituitary adenomas

Plurihormonal pituitary adenomas are defined as tumors that show immunoreactivity for more than one hormone that cannot be explained by normal cytophysiology or developmental mechanism [5]. They can be monomorphous, consisting of a single cell type producing two or more hormones, or plurimorphous, consisting of two or more different cell lineages.

Plurihormonality is reported in the literature; it is estimated rare in most studied series while they are more frequent in other series [5, 6–8]. Most plurihormonal adenomas are silent [2]. Various combinations are described in the literature in the studied series:

- PRL and LH; PRL and TSH [7]
- GH and ACTH [9–11]
- PRL and ACTH [5, 7, 12, 13]
- ACTH, LH, and TSH [7]
- PRL, LH, FSH, and TSH [7]
- GH, PRL, TSH, and a-SU [5]
- GH, PRL, and ACTH [7, 14]
- GH, PRL, TSH, FSH, and aSU [15]

Other less common combinations are also published [5]. Original examples of plurihormonal adenomas in the author series [7] are shown in **Figures 1–3**.

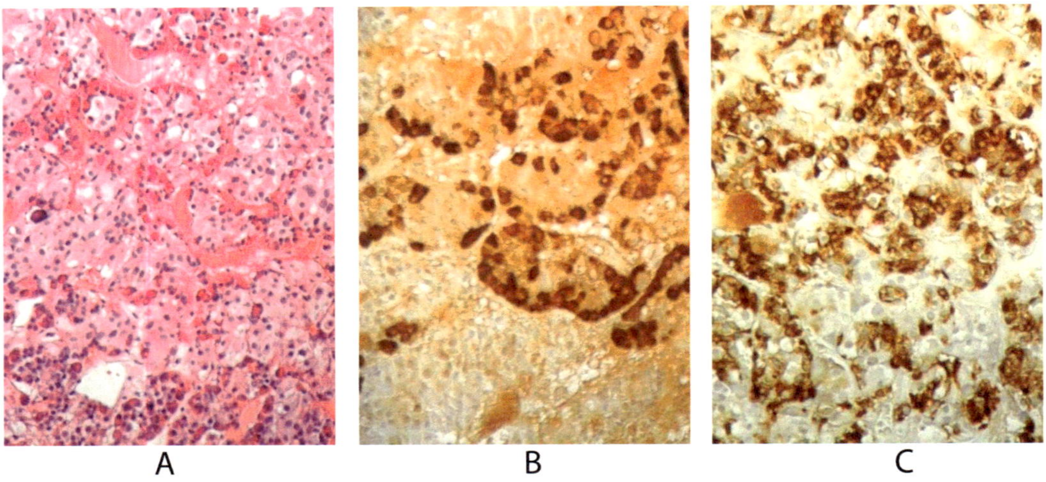

Figure 1. (A) Pituitary adenoma revealing a trabecular and nested structure (HE stain, x200), composed of two distinct types of cells. (B) ACTH secretion in the same adenoma (x400, ACTH-antibody, Dako). (C) Prolactin secretion in the same adenoma (x400, PRL-antibody, Dako). Positive stain is demonstrated in different cells than cells positive for ACTH. Detection of other pituitary hormones was negative.

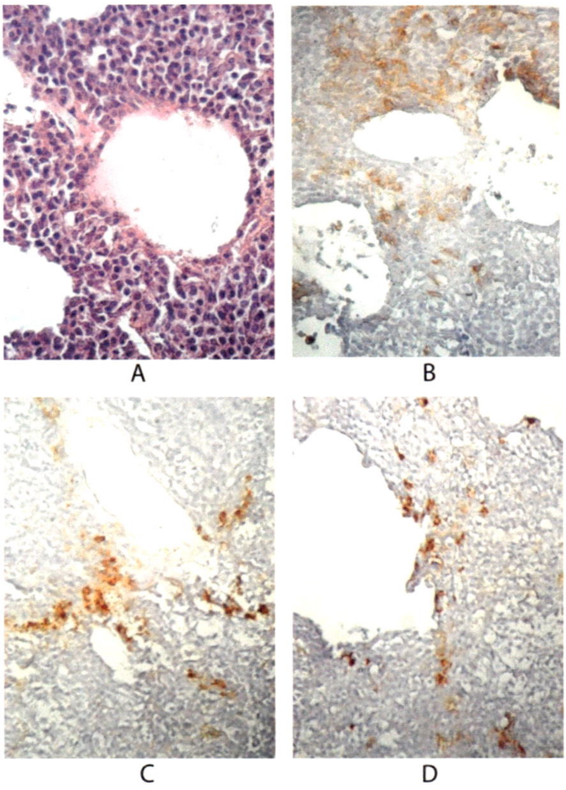

Figure 2. (A) Pituitary adenoma revealing a pseudoglandular and microcystic structure (x400, HE stain). (B). Prolactin secretion in some tumor cells (x400, PRL-antibody, Dako). (C) TSH secretion in the same tumor, apparently in different cells than prolactin secretion (x400, TSH-antibody, Dako). (D) FSH secretion in the same tumor, apparently in different cells than prolactin and TSH secretion (x400, FSH-antibody, Dako).

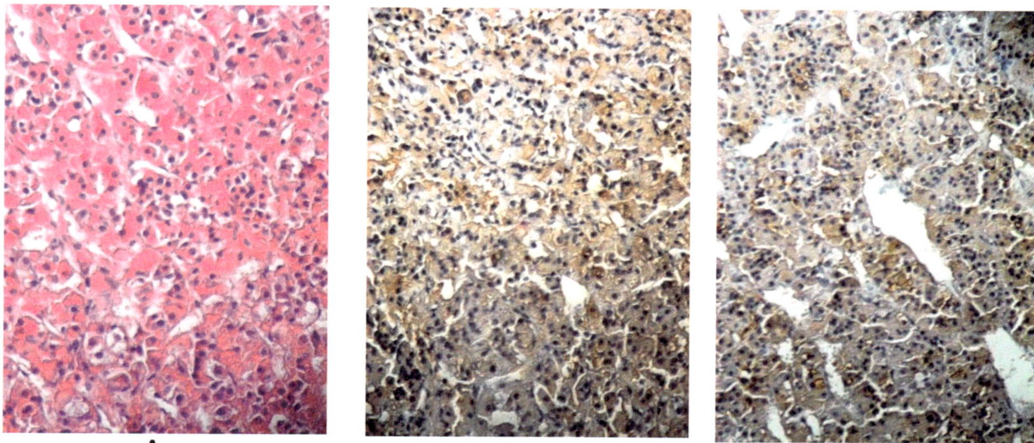

Figure 3. (A) Crooke cell adenoma (x400, HE stain). (B) ACTH secretion in the same Crooke cell adenoma (x400, ACTH-antibody, Dako). (C). Prolactin secretion in the same crook cell adenoma, apparently positive in the same cells as ACTH (x400, PRL-antibody, Dako). Detection of other pituitary hormones was negative.

Some of the secretions might remain subclinical and only detected by immunohistochemical studies.

It was noted that half of the somatotroph adenomas, particularly densely granulated adenomas, secrete other hormones; these hormones are not clinically relevant [1, 3].

A combination of hormone secretion was also reported in double pituitary adenoma base on two separate tumors on MRI imaging or histopathologic examination [5].

Pituitary adenomas with the combination of different hormone groups from the same cell lineage (GH and prolactin or FSH and LH) are relatively common, but true plurihormonal adenomas with immunoreactivities that cross the cytogenetic lineage are rare in most series as "in Refs. [5, 6, 13]."

The challenging points are:

1. How many cells that are positive for each type of hormones or pituitary transcription factors can allow the diagnosis of plurihormonal adenoma?

2. The new definition of the null cell adenoma requires the demonstration of immunonegativity for pituitary transcription factors and adenohypophyseal hormones [2, 16]; however, does the observation of rare or few positive cells for immunohistochemical markers allow to rule out the diagnosis of null cell adenoma?

4. Hormone secretion and prognosis of pituitary adenomas

Many studies tried to find out the criteria for predicting the prognosis and development of pituitary adenomas; though most of them have benign outcomes, others might have adverse outcomes and be able to invade locally, resist conventional therapy, or might recur or metastasize [2].

The following question is raised: Is any relationships exist between hormone secretion and prognosis of pituitary adenomas?

4.1. Potentially "aggressive pituitary adenoma"

Certain subtypes of pituitary adenomas are found tending to show more aggressive clinical behavior and designed by some authors as aggressive adenomas [2]; these are: sparsely granulated somatotroph adenoma (SGSA), lactotroph macroadenoma in men, Crooke cell adenoma, silent corticotroph adenoma, and plurihormonal PIT1-positive adenoma (previously called silent subtype 3 adenomas [1–3, 5]). It is also reported that pituitary adenomas found in MEN1 (multiple endocrine neoplasia type 1) tend to be plurihormonal and more aggressive [12].

4.2. "High-risk pituitary adenoma"

The defined criteria for this adenoma in the last 4th WHO classification for pituitary adenomas are, as "in Refs. [2, 3, 17]":

- Rapid growth
- Radiological invasion
- High Ki-67 proliferation index more than 3%

This adenoma tends to predict recurrence and resistance to conventional therapy [2].

It is not clear whether all potentially "aggressive pituitary adenomas" are "high-risk adenomas," as the first term depends on hormone secretion, while the second term depends on clinical and radiological data plus the immunohistochemical study for Ki-67 proliferation index. P53 is not considered as an independent risk factor [2].

A high risk adenoma with histological signs of aggressiveness is shown in **Figure 4**.

4.3. "Atypical adenoma"

The term "atypical adenoma" was previously used in the 3rd WHO classification [1]; it is defined by a high mitotic index, Ki-67 mitotic index more than 3%, and strong nuclear P53 staining. This term is no more used in the 4th classification [2], as it did not prove any utility. Atypical adenoma is replaced by the definition of "high-risk adenoma." Strong positive nuclear expression of P53 is not proved to be an independent factor of high-risk adenoma [2].

4.4. Plurihormonality and prognosis

Plurihormonal PIT1-positive adenomas are aggressive in terms of their size, growth rate, and invasiveness, with cavernous sinus invasion occurring in 67% of cases and 31% rate of recurrence [5].

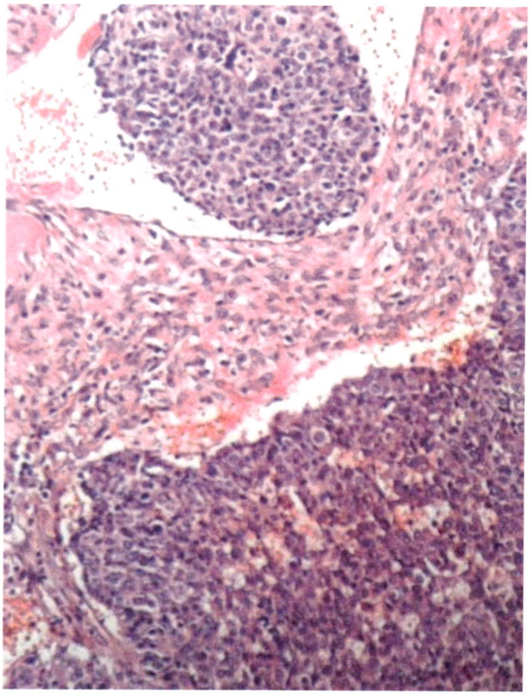

Figure 4. Aggressive and high-risk pituitary adenoma revealing vascular invasion and mitotic figures (x200, HE stain). It demonstrated immunonegativity for hormone secretion.

4.5. Pituitary carcinoma

The only conclusive criterion of malignancy is actually metastasis. The last WHO classification of pituitary adenomas strictly defined pituitary carcinoma as a tumor of adenohypophyseal cells that metastasizes craniospinally or is associated with systemic metastasis. This definition is independent of the histological appearance; as histologically, about 60% of primary tumors have features of a conventional adenoma [2, 18].

Pre-metastatic lesions and metastases can be hormonally active or clinically nonfunctioning. There are no clinical or biochemical features specific to an adenoma that will metastasize [18]. No confirmed relationship is demonstrated between non-secreting adenoma, plurihormonality, and malignancy; though, plurihormonal PIT1-positive carcinomas have also been reported [18].

4.6. Pituitary neuroendocrine tumor (PitNET)

This term is recently proposed in 2017 for pituitary adenoma by the International Pituitary Pathology Club to explain the highly variable clinical impact of pituitary adenomas on patients and the poor reproducibility of the actual predictive markers [19] though the margins are not clear between pituitary adenomas and neuroendocrine tumors.

Pituitary carcinomas are demonstrated positive for neuroendocrine differentiation like synaptophysin and chromogranin A [18].

5. Necessity of hormone detection by immunohistochemical studies

5.1. Questions frequently raised when we have a case of pituitary adenoma

Pathologists and clinicians might ask the following questions:

1. Is it necessary to make histological study to every pituitary adenoma?
2. Is it necessary to demonstrate hormonal production in all pituitary adenomas studied by pathologists?
3. How many antibodies should a pathologist use to study this adenoma?
4. Which antibodies have clinical utility for treatment and prognostic prediction?
5. Can we predict the aggressiveness of a pituitary adenoma before that it becomes clinically and radiologically aggressive?

5.2. Importance of immunohistochemical studies

We might find answers on the previous questions in the following findings:

- Classification of pituitary adenomas requires morphological and hormonal immunohistochemical assessment [2, 3].
- Nonfunctional adenomas, with no hormone detection in the serum, are not necessarily nonproducing adenomas. Detection of hormonal production by immunostaining leads to term them "silent adenomas" [2, 3]. Some authors recently proposed to term them "poorly differentiated Pit-1 lineage adenomas" [20].
- Immunostaining is important to diagnose some of the potentially "aggressive adenomas" subtypes as mentioned before.
- Detection of PIT1 and hormonal production is important for the diagnosis of plurihormonal PIT1-positive pituitary adenomas (previously called silent subtype 3 adenomas) that are considered as potentially "aggressive adenoma" [2, 5].
- Detection of the somatostatin receptor by immunohistochemistry may be a useful predictor of treatment response, as SGSAs are less responsive to somatostatin antagonists and may require treatment with the GH receptor antagonist pegvisomant [21].
- Demonstration of immunonegativity for hormones and transcription factors, especially Pit-1, is important for the differential diagnosis between silent adenomas and null cell adenoma, as the latter has good prognosis. Some silent adenomas, notably silent corticotroph adenoma and plurihormonal PIT1-positive adenoma (previously called silent subtype 3 adenomas), are considered potentially "aggressive adenomas" [2, 17, 22].

- Demonstration of NSE, chromogranin A and synaptophysin helps to diagnose PitNET and might predict more aggressive potential even before that the tumor comes clinically and radiologically aggressive.

5.3. Recommended antibodies for the diagnosis and prediction

It is important to demonstrate hormone production, transcription factors for functional differentiation, and proliferation index that indicate prediction. Practically, the following immunohistochemical stains are recommended in studying a pituitary adenoma as they cover wide area of diagnosis and prediction:

- GH, prolactin, TSH-beta, ACTH, FSH-beta, LH-beta, and alpha-SU to make an accurate classification of the studied pituitary adenoma.
- Pit-1 and TPIT transcription factors and ER-alpha are recommended when there is immunonegativity for pituitary hormones, to rule out potentially aggressive silent adenomas. SF1, the transcription factor for gonadotroph cell lineage does not seem to have prognostic importance, as gonadotroph adenomas are usually not aggressive.
- Ki-67 proliferation index, for the demonstration of "high-risk adenomas."
- Chromogranin A and synaptophysin diagnose PitNET that might predict more aggressive behavior.
- P53 is not an independent risk factor of aggressiveness; so it is not necessary to demonstrate it.

6. Conclusions

Immunohistochemical studies have increasing importance in pituitary adenomas. Demonstration of hormones, some transcription factors and cofactors for functional differentiation, and proliferation index have important roles in the classification, prediction, and treatment of these adenomas, as demonstration of neuroendocrine differentiation.

Conflict of interest

I declare that there is no "conflict of interest" in this chapter.

Author details

Raydeh Al Khani

Address all correspondence to: raydeh.alkhani@gmail.com

Professor of Pathology, Faculty of Medicine, Damascus University, Damascus, Syria

References

[1] Lloyd RV, Kovacs K, Young WF Jr, Farrell W, Asa SL, et al. Pituitary tumors: Introduction. In: Delellis RA, Lloyd RV, Heitz PU, Eng C, editors. World Health Organization Classification of Tumors. Pathology and Genetics of Tumors of Endocrine Organs. 3rd ed. Lyon: IARC Press; 2004

[2] Osamura RY, Lopes MBS, Grossman A, Kontogeorgos G, Trouillas J. Introduction. In: Lloyd RV, Osamura RY, Klöppel G, Rosai J. editors. World Health Organization Classification of Tumors. WHO Classification of Tumours of Endocrine Organs. 4th ed. IARC Press: Lyon 2017. pp. 13

[3] Osamura RY, Grossman A, Korbonits M, Kovacs K, Lopes MBS, et al. Pituitary adenoma. In: Lloyd RV, Osamura RY, Klöppel G, Rosai J, editors. World Health Organization Classification of Tumors. WHO Classification of Tumours of Endocrine Organs. 4th ed. Lyon: IARC Press; 2017. pp. 14-18

[4] Nishioka H, Inoshita N, Mete O, Asa SL, Hayashi K, et al. The complementary role of transcription factors in the accurate diagnosis of clinically nonfunctioning pituitary adenomas. Endocrine Pathology. 2015;**26**:349-355. DOI: 10.1007/s12022-015-9398-z

[5] Kontogeorgos G, Kovacs K, Lloyd RV, Righi A. Plurihormonal and double adenoma. In: Lloyd RV, Osamura RY, Klöppel G, Rosai J, editors. World Health Organization Classification of Tumors. WHO Classification of Tumours of Endocrine Organs. 4th ed. Lyon: IARC Press; 2017. pp. 39-40

[6] Saeger W, Lüdecke DK, Buchfelder M, Fahlbusch R, Quabbe HJ, Petersenn S. Pathohistological classification of pituitary tumors: 10 years of experience with the German Pituitary Tumor Registry. European Journal of Endocrinology. 2007;**156**(2): 203-216. DOI: 10.1530/eje.1.02326

[7] Al Khani R. Plurihormonal secretion in pituitary adenomas: Immunohistological study of 100 cases. JABMS (Journal of the Arab Board of Medical Specializations). 2002;**4**(4): 89-95E. ISSN 1561-0217

[8] Kwinta BM, Krzyżewski RM, Kliś K, Adamek D. Quantitative immunohistochemical assessment of clinically non-functioning pituitary adenomas. Medical Research Journal. 2017;**2**(4):147-151. DOI: 10.5603/MRJ.2017.0020

[9] Rajendran R, Naik S, Sandeman DD, Nasruddin AB. Pasireotide therapy in a rare and unusual case of plurihormonal pituitary macroadenoma. Endocrinology, Diabetes & Metabolism Case Reports. 2013;**2013**:130026. DOI: 10.1530/EDM-13-0026

[10] Rasul FT, Jaunmuktane Z, Khan AA, Phadke R, Powell M. Plurihormonal pituitary adenoma with concomitant adrenocorticotropic hormone (ACTH) and growth hormone (GH) secretion: A report of two cases and review of the literature. Acta Neurochirurgica. 2014;**156**(1):141-146. DOI: 10.1007/s00701-013-1890-y

[11] Roca E, Mattogno PP, Porcelli T, Poliani L, Belotti F, et al. Plurihormonal ACTH-GH pituitary adenoma: Case report and systematic literature review. World Neurosurgery. 2018;**114**:e158-e164. DOI: 10.1016/j.wneu.2018.02.120

[12] Uraki S, Ariyasu H, Doi A, Furuta H, Nishi M, et al. Hypersecretion of ACTH and PRL from pituitary adenoma in MEN1, adequately managed by medical therapy. Endocrinology, Diabetes & Metabolism Case Reports. 2017;**2017**:17-0027. Published online 2017 Apr 6. DOI: 10.1530/EDM-17-0027

[13] Kunasegaran S, Croxson MS, Holdaway I, Murphy R. An unusual case of Cushing's syndrome due to bihormonal ACTH–prolactin secreting pituitary macroadenoma with rapid response to cabergoline. https://www.ncbi.nlm.nih.gov/pubmed/28784879. BMJ case reports. BMJ Case Reports. 2017 Aug 7;2017. DOI: 10.1136/bcr-2017-219921

[14] Batisse Lignier M, Maqdasy S, Mestre B, Roche B, Chazal J, Tauveron I. An unusual plurihormonal pituitary adenoma. In: 15th International & 14th European Congress of Endocrinology; 05-09 May 2012; Florence, Italy. Endocrine Abstracts; 2012; 29. p. 1540

[15] Luk CT, Kovacs K, Rotondo F, Horvath E, Cusimano M, Booth GL. Plurihormonal pituitary adenoma immunoreactive for thyroid-stimulating hormone, growth hormone, follicle-stimulating hormone, and prolactin. Endocrine Practice. 2012;**18**(5):e121-e126. DOI: 10.4158/EP12033.CR

[16] Mete O, Lopes MB. Overview of the 2017 WHO Classification of Pituitary Tumors. Endocrine Pathology. 2017;**28**(3):228-243. DOI: 10.1007/s12022-017-9498-z

[17] Nishioka H, Inoshita N. New WHO classification of pituitary adenomas (4th edition): Assessment of pituitary transcription factors and the prognostic histological factors. Brain Tumor Pathology. 2018;**35**(2):57-61. DOI: 10.1007/s10014-017-0307-7

[18] Roncaroli F, Kovacs K, Lloyd RV, Matsuno A, Righi A. Pituitary carcinoma. In: Lloyd RV, Osamura RY, Klöppel G, Rosai J, editors. World Health Organization Classification of Tumors. WHO Classification of Tumours of Endocrine Organs. 4th ed. Lyon: IARC Press; 2017. pp. 41-44

[19] Asa SL, Casar-Borota O, Chanson P, Delgrange E, Earls P, et al. From pituitary adenoma to pituitary neuroendocrine tumor (PitNET): An International Pituitary Pathology Club proposal. Endocrine-Related Cancer. 2017;**24**(4):C5-C8. DOI: 10.1530/ERC-17-0004

[20] Mete O, Gomez-Hernandez K, Kucharczyk W, Ridout R, Zadeh G, et al. Silent subtype 3 pituitary adenomas are not always silent and represent poorly differentiated monomorphous plurihormonal Pit-1 lineage adenomas. Modern Pathology. 2016;**29**(2):131-142. DOI: 10.1038/modpathol.2015.151

[21] Mete O, Korbonits M, Osamura RY, Trouillas J, Yamada S. Somatotroph adenoma. In: Lloyd RV, Osamura RY, Klöppel G, Rosai J, editors. World Health Organization Classification of Tumors. WHO Classification of Tumours of Endocrine Organs. 4th ed. Lyon: IARC Press; 2017. pp. 19-23

[22] Lee JC, Pekmezci M, Lavezo JL, Vogel H, Katznelson L, et al. Utility of Pit-1 immunostaining in distinguishing pituitary adenomas of primitive differentiation from null cell adenomas. Endocrine Pathology. 2017;**28**(4):287-292. DOI: 10.1007/s12022-017-9503-6